"Bravo! Adele has magnificently captured years of work and experience in a sound and complete program. This book clearly identifies the emotional, behavioral, and physiological aspects that contribute to overeating and weight gain. With compassion and tenderness this book offers tools and insights to successfully deal with all aspects of overeating. Adele has combined all the right ingredients so that the readers come away learning how to be good to themselves, take care of their minds and bodies, and lose weight in the process."
— SONDRA KRONBERG, M.S., R.D., C.N.
    President of the Eating Disorder Council of
    Long Island

"Once you start with Adele Puhn's program, you're in it for life. Weight-loss and fitness programs come and go, but Adele's unique approach really works! In some ways it's like magic. Not only do you lose weight, but you feel incredibly better. And it's an easy plan to live with because it becomes part of your everyday routine; I recommend it heartily."
— PHIL DUSENBERRY
    Chairman of the Board, BBDO

"After years of failure with nutrition plans and diets that included pills and injections, I have found a new lifestyle thanks to Adele Puhn's nutrition plan. My blood sugar is good, my weight is substantially less, and I have considerably more energy and vitality. I have truly found a new way of living."

    —CARL LEVINE
      Former Vice President of
      Bloomingdale's Department Stores

"Adele's system organizes not only a sensible way of eating but also a sensible way of living."

    —GLENN DUBOSE
      Managing Director
      Cultural and Arts Programs, Thirteen/WNET

By Adele Puhn
Published by Ballantine Books:

THE 5-DAY MIRACLE DIET
THE 5-DAY MIRACLE DIET COMPANION

THE 5-DAY MIRACLE DIET

CONQUER FOOD CRAVINGS,
LOSE WEIGHT, AND FEEL BETTER
THAN YOU EVER HAVE
IN YOUR LIFE!

Adele Puhn, M.S., C.N.S.

BALLANTINE BOOKS • NEW YORK

http://www.randomhouse.com

Library of Congress Catalog Card Number: 96-95271

ISBN 0-345-41998-7

Manufactured in the United States of America

First Hardcover Edition: May 1996
First Mass Market Edition: May 1997

10 9 8 7 6 5 4 3 2 1

This book is dedicated with the deepest love to my dearest friend— my husband, Arthur.

CONTENTS

ACKNOWLEDGMENTS

During the many years it took to develop this program and write the *The 5-Day Miracle Diet*, I have been surrounded by many loving and supportive people. I am particularly grateful to my husband, Arthur, whose constant support, belief, and love enabled me to travel the road that led to the completion of this book. I thank him for his patience and his availability, and for endless hours of reading, editing, and discussion. Most of all, I thank him for being there at the beginning.

My apologies and thanks to my loving children, Bonnee and David, who endured the early years of experimentation long before the *New Nutrition* was practiced, for the times they spent having vitamins and Twinkie-less parties, for Halloweens with raisins and natural whole grain cookies instead of the sugar-coated chocolate-dipped ones they would rather have had. But I now delightfully reap the rewards of having fostered this nutritional awareness when I see my three-year-old granddaughter Charlotte munch on carrot sticks instead of lollipops. I trust that my two just-born grandchildren, Lindsay and Jake, will be doing the same. I also want my son-in-law Danny and daughter-in-law Melissa to know that I appreciate their continued love, support, and heartfelt excitement. And I offer my sympathies to my stepdaughters, Alyson and Margot, for years of eating veggies and stir fry instead of Big Macs and SpaghettiOs which they, like other young children, would have preferred.

Special thanks go to my agent, Wendy Weil, who saw the strength of my program and the potential of *The 5-Day Miracle Diet* even before it was written. Her help was the first step in making this book a reality.

I am indebted to Karla Dougherty, whose help and writing talents enabled me to transform this "book in my head" onto the written page. Her ability to put my thoughts and words into a cohesive and presentable format helped make this book what it is.

I am indebted to Ballantine Books for their ardent support of this book and individually want to thank editor-in-chief Joëlle Delbourgo, who had the insight to understand my program and bring this book to being. To editor Elizabeth Zack, who enthusiastically carried the flame, I give my heartfelt thanks. I am grateful to the entire staff at Ballantine whose guidance and talents helped to shape this book into its final state. President Linda Grey gave strong support and publisher Clare Ferraro offered reassurance in times of need. To publicists Kim Hovey and Jennifer Richards, art director Ruth Ross, and all the other wonderful Ballantine people, your constant excitement was used as fuel to keep my energy high. Thank you!

To my dear friend Donna Gellman I want to express my deepest appreciation for her creation of the "Fifteen-Minute Stretch," and her encouragement, support, and sharing of her special talents. To Susanna Weiss, trainer extraordinaire, a grateful thanks for the time and energy spent on the exercise chapter.

A successful career does not get built by one individual alone. Along the way I've had the good fortune to work with knowledgeable, caring professionals. I want to express my deepest appreciation to Dr. Evelyn Leigner, whose professional supervision continues to enlighten me and enhance the work I do; Dr. Charles Goodrich, whose early recognition of my work encouraged me at a time when the medical profession did not "believe"; Dr. Shari Leiberman, nutritionist and friend, who encouraged me to take the time from a busy practice to write; and Maria Schestopalow, my secretary, who, with her usual good nature, kept the office humming in spite of the increased workload created by the writing of this book. I also thank Dr. Richard Ash for his generosity in both time and support; chiropractors Dr. Nancy Brand, Dr. Sally Brooke-Smith, and masseuse Jane Factor for their physical and emotional support when the going was the toughest; and the staff at Navona, my favorite local restaurant, for the wonderful lunches that kept my blood sugar balanced, enabling me to keep focused on my writing.

Special words of appreciation go to my attorney, Michael Rudell, who demonstrated his faith in *The 5-Day Miracle Diet* by introducing me to my literary agent, and to Jo Sgammato and Ponchitta Pierce, who offered me the benefit of their expertise in the publishing field.

I want to say a special thanks to my brother and sister-in-law, Marty and Mary Green, for their enthusiastic advice, and to the friends who have listened to my ideas during busy times, giving support and suggestions throughout this process: Ellie Dubin, Dr. Susan Hans, Sondra Kronberg, R.D., C.N.S., Maxine Pines, Lenore Rauch, Ellie Rothchild, M.S.W., and Margery Weinroth. Thanks also to my mother-in-law Sydelle Prince, whose loving support was greatly felt.

And these acknowledgments would never be complete or even possible without the support, encouragement, and thoughtful help of my many clients. Indeed there would be no program without their willingness to explore the new and unknown. It was these experiences over the years that allowed me to define and redefine the program as you see it today. I want to thank each and every one of them for providing the rich source of material that allowed me to turn this program into *The 5-Day Miracle Diet*.

As with any diet and exercise program, please confer with your health professional before starting the 5-Day Miracle Diet plan—especially if you are taking any medications on a regular basis.

THE 5-DAY MIRACLE DIET

I Was Born in a Box of Cookies

Put aside every notion you ever had about diets. Toss out your food pyramids, your low-fat cookies, your bananas, and your carbo-packed breakfasts, lunches, and dinners.

And while you're at it, throw away words such as *will-power*, *motivation*, *cravings*, and *urges*.

You are about to begin a new way of life. You will feel fabulous on a day-to-day basis—and lose weight, too.

Within the pages of this book you will learn about a food program so innovative, so exciting, and so effective that you will never have to "diet" again.

CONFESSIONS OF A FOOD SENSUALIST

My 5-Day Miracle Diet did not happen by accident. I did not conjure up the idea one night in my sleep and simply offer it to my clients the next morning. No. It took twenty years of experience, of trial and error, of exhaustive research and experimentation, of thought and forethought, for me to devise a plan that, even today, is being refined and defined to fit every individual situation.

It began at home, with my overweight mother's mixed signals. "Don't eat too much or you'll look like me," she would say as she brought home the cookies, the Danish, and the freshly baked jelly doughnuts. I might not have

1

wanted to follow in the footsteps of my mother (or my diabetic father, for that matter), but at the same time I could not resist those tantalizing white bakery bags. The "Green genes" (my maiden name) had taken root long before I was a newborn babe. I was preordained to be a food sensualist. You might say I was born in a cookie box.

I began to eat—and I did not stop until graduate school.

Oh, sure, I tried diets—one after another, like everyone else. Diet pills, Weight Watchers, Stillman's, Atkins, Schmatikins—you name it and I did it. And I even had success; I lost weight—for a while. But soon my sweet tooth overcame my white-knuckled willpower.

I needed a cookie.

In fact there were moments when I needed a cookie more than anything else in my entire life.

That cookie represented love, power, control, and happiness.

And I know I'm not alone.

IT ALL COMES DOWN TO CHEMISTRY

"There were times when nothing existed in the world except me and that cookie. I *had* to have it."

"When I start eating pasta, I can't stop. I can go through an entire box!"

"Every afternoon I crave a chocolate bar. I have to have it. But it doesn't really help. Forty-five minutes later I'm ready for a nap."

"I don't know. I can't focus. I'm depressed. I'm not really hungry, but I want to eat."

"I've tried everything—and I still can't lose weight."

These are all comments I have heard from my clients. Indeed, they are all comments I have said myself.

Wait a minute. Losing weight and keeping it off should not be an impossible feat. You don't have to accept your weight—or that sluggish, tired, depressed feeling that frequently accompanies those extra pounds.

I knew there had to be more to my cravings than that "cookie box cradle"—especially when I saw my son, David, also exhibit low-blood-sugar cravings and behaviors. He was seven years old when a doctor diagnosed him as being hyperactive. He was bright, active, and articulate—but he was unable to stand still.

Dr. Feingold's theories about sugar as a cause of hyperactivity were just becoming known at the time. My interest in nutrition led me to his books. I read everything I could find. I did an enormous amount of research and observation; after all, this was my son. I watched David and noticed that the more cookies he had, the more he wanted. And the more sugar he ate, the more cranky, unfocused, and hyperactive he became. I could recognize when he had eaten candy at a friend's house. He would storm into the house, shouting and running up and down the stairs, ready for another sugar "hit." He would jump in place and literally cry for a cookie. The chemical "hook" was definitely at work; he was a totally different boy than the calmer one—crisp, healthy apple in hand—who had left a few hours earlier to play.

I wanted to help my son—and I didn't want to do it with medication. I realized that when he was not eating candy or cookies, he was more focused and his energy level was where it should be for a healthy, active (but not hyperactive) seven-year-old. I knew there had to be a connection between the sugar he ate and the way he behaved, and I was determined to find out exactly what that connection was.

By the time I reached graduate school, I had the tools I needed to discover the answers to my questions. I knew there was a definite connection between blood-sugar levels, cravings, and behavior. It was just a matter of time until I learned what has become a mission—for David, for myself, and for everyone who thinks more about cookies than living a full, productive life.

While I was writing a master's thesis on biochemistry and science, I used my earlier training in library science to advantage, trying to find out why that cookie was so important.

I was interning at a holistic clinic while attending school; I was intrigued by the "alternative" medicines its health professionals used, preventative measures such as shiatsu massage, vitamins, and herbal teas that today are considered commonplace. I was open to new ideas—and I was smart enough to know that the "cookie monster," even for a seven-year-old, was too powerful to be the product of pure thought.

Our cravings for a cookie had to have a physical base. It felt like a jolt, a drop-dead, hold-me-down, fight-or-flight physiological arousal. Pure and simple, I realized that our food cravings—and yours—are a physical need. And like breathing or fighting for survival, needs always win hands down.

And that's when, in a particularly late session at the library in 1979, the 5-Day Miracle Diet was born, a program that combines different foods with different textures eaten at different times to manipulate the body—and its blood-sugar levels.

Sixteen years later I have a master's in medical biology and clinical nutrition from the University of Bridgeport. I have earned the title of Certified Nutrition Specialist (CNS) awarded by the American College of Nutrition, a prestigious association composed of medical and research specialists whose main purpose is to further nutrition research. I have taught classes in consumer awareness and lectured extensively for important groups such as the American Cancer Society and the United Jewish Appeal. I maintain a private practice in Manhattan and Great Neck, working on a referral basis with many doctors, specialists, psychotherapists, psychiatrists, and even restaurateurs.

In short I've been around, and I've learned a few important truths.

Losing weight and keeping it off has nothing to do with willpower.

It has nothing to do with deprivation.

It has nothing to do with low-fat cookies, cheeses, meat, dressings, sauces, or any other member of the low-fat food group.

It has nothing to do with outsmarting those fat cells that supposedly cry out, like the infamous plant in the classic film *Little Shop of Horrors*, "Feed me. . . ."

And, for most people, it has nothing to do with the roll they had at lunch.

Losing weight and keeping it off is largely dependent on stable blood-sugar levels.

More specifically, *preventing low blood sugar and creating a state of good blood sugar.*

THERE'S NOTHING LIKE THE FEELING OF WELL-BEING, THE ENERGY, AND THE VITALITY THAT COME FROM LIVING IN GOOD BLOOD SUGAR—NOT TO MENTION THE DELIGHT AS YOUR WEIGHT DROPS OFF!

Most of us live in low blood sugar. It's true. A glucose tolerance test might not show that you're hypoglycemic, but you might as well be. The way you eat, the types of food you eat, and the times you eat—all these factors make for highs and lows the whole day through. Indeed, if you were to test your blood throughout a twenty-four-hour period, you'd find those highs and lows that produce hypoglycemic symptoms.

Take away the low-blood-sugar levels in your body and you will lose the physiological cravings for starches, sweets, alcohol, caffeine, and fats. You will have more energy than you have ever had in your life. You will be more focused and experience a greater sense of well-being than you've ever thought possible.

In actuality 75 percent of the reason why you cannot lose weight and keep it off is physiological. It's the low blood sugar that keeps those cravings coming.

The other 25 percent is what I call *the fathead*: the behaviors, feelings, and psychological underpinnings that, combined with low blood sugar, keep you fat.

Listen:

THE ACCOUNTANT AND THE CHOCOLATE CAKE

One of my clients, an accountant in his late fifties, was going to a family gathering over the weekend. While discussing the week ahead during our session, he decided he did not want to deviate from the 5-Day Miracle Diet one iota. He had already lost twenty-two pounds and was in excellent blood sugar. He was eager to reach his goal weight and wanted to be "perfect." I urged him to relax, to enjoy the party, and even to allow himself some extra food. He knew, as do all my clients, that if he decided to eat something in addition to the basic diet plan, it was absolutely fine. (In fact, it's imperative at least once a week. But it has to be something *fabulous*, something you *adore*, something you want above all else.) Even knowing all this, my client shook his head no. He wanted to get to his goal as soon as possible.

He was ripe for sabotage. As he came through the

door, all his relatives oohed and aahed at his weight loss. His favorite aunt was there with open arms. "There you are! You look great! And guess what? I've made your favorite chocolate cake."

He did not stop to think. He could not escape. In fact because he had not prepared himself to eat something extra, he didn't have a clue as to how to deal with his aunt and her cake. He had not planned any strategies. He had not analyzed the situations that might have come up. The moral? He not only ate one piece, he ate three pieces— unable to enjoy one single bite. With every forkful of cake he felt rage—at his aunt and at himself. He didn't even love the chocolate cake! It was a myth perpetuated by the family to make his aunt feel loved and admired.

Coupled with the guilt that inevitably followed the last piece he polished off, he sealed his fate. He went home and continued to eat. He ate all week. It was a vicious cycle. The lower his blood sugar, the more he craved his sweets—anything to fill the need. The more sweets he ate, the more he stayed in bad blood sugar. Worse, the more he ate, the more he felt "fat, ugly, and disgusting." The result? He continued to eat, making his "fat, ugly, and disgusting" persona a self-fulfilling prophecy. The cycle was in place—just as it had been for me, for my son, and very possibly the way it has continued to be for you.

The 5-Day Miracle Diet will change all that.

Call it a wonder. Call it a miracle. Whatever, it's . . .

THE ONLY DIET BOOK YOU'LL EVER NEED— OR WANT—AGAIN

Within the pages of *The 5-Day Miracle Diet*, the work has been done for you. The calculations and the research, the experimentation and the analysis, have been finely tuned, making the program easy and simple to follow. All you have to do is follow the 5-Day Miracle Diet for five days and you will "miraculously" lose the cravings, the urges, that make you want to overeat. Once you've lost the physiological needs that are 75 percent of your problem, I will show you how to deal with the remaining 25 percent. This makes up your *fathead*, including advice and strategies to resist the saboteurs: the people around you, your family and friends, and even yourself, especially the "eating of your feelings" that, like the accountant and his chocolate cake, we are all so compelled to do. I will even provide a quiz to help you see if you are one of the segment of the overweight population that is carbohydrate addicted; I will show you how to modify my program to *strip the carbs* without creating a feeling of deprivation.

The proof is in the doing. Follow the 5-Day Miracle Diet and you will see how, less and less, your body craves those sweets, those starches, or that bottle of Chardonnay. It will show you how you can have your cake—and eat it, too.

Now, at last, you can control your body—instead of it controlling you.

A POUND OF CURE: LOSING WEIGHT AND HYPERTENSION, TOO

For every two pounds a person loses, his or her blood pressure is also reduced by one millimeter of mercury.

A CLIENT'S TALE

I remember the day Ellie first came into my office. It was spring. The sun was beaming through my sheer-curtained windows; a light breeze brushed the papers on my desk.

The three clients I'd seen before her had been imbued with optimism. They couldn't help it. Just walking outside had lifted their spirits. It was a beautiful day.

I'd spoken to Ellie only briefly on the phone a few days before to set up our appointment. She'd been referred by another client, a colleague at the pharmaceutical firm where she worked as an account executive. Ellie's problem was similar to ones I've heard over and over again in my practice: She kept losing and gaining the same twenty pounds. She couldn't keep the weight off, and now that she was in her forties, the weight was staying put—and climbing. Worse, her cholesterol levels and blood pressure were creeping into serious numbers.

Ellie was overweight, but she was attractive. She had achieved some financial and professional success. She had a child, a nine-year-old daughter from a previous marriage, a steady beau, and a wide circle of friends. There seemed no apparent reason for her mood, but she was still depressed. More than depressed. She was lethargic, out of focus, and full of self-loathing. Why couldn't she lose weight!!!!

We started to get to know each other during that first session. We discussed her eating habits, the orange juice and cereal she always had for breakfast, the pasta dishes for lunch, and the bananas and no-fat frozen yogurt she had for snacks. I knew these habits needed to be changed, so I immediately put her on the 5-Day Miracle Diet. Over the ensuing months I modified it to meet her needs—as you, too, will learn to do in this book. Like some of my other clients, she was skeptical at first. "That's it? This is all I have to do?"

I nodded. "Trust me."

She did. Within five months Ellie had lost thirty-five pounds. She felt wonderful; she had more energy than she had had in years. Her cholesterol and blood pressure were down and she looked terrific.

Now I say to you, trust me. Read what I have to say. And you, too, will learn what Ellie and all my other clients have learned about their bodies' physiological needs and the sabotage that goes on in their minds. You, too, can begin the journey toward a healthier, happier life.

A STORY I TELL MY CLIENTS

Several years after I began to develop what became the 5-Day Miracle Diet, I was at a friend's holiday party. There were dozens of people there: grandparents, friends, parents, children, teens, toddlers, babies, even a couple of dogs. My friend had had her first child six months earlier. The baby was just learning to stand up. There she was, in the living room, surrounded by adults sitting on couches and chairs, all of them eating (of course), drinking, and laughing. She got up on her tiny legs . . . and immediately fell down, more frightened than hurt.

Understandably the little girl cried. And cried. Within twenty seconds her father ran over to her, and with the finesse of a tennis pro lobbing a brilliant serve, he lifted her up in one hand while simultaneously reaching for a cookie with the other.

The girl stopped crying.

In that brief period she learned four things about life:

- It's not okay to cry. Emotions are scary and best over with quickly.
- Any emotion, from pain to bliss, however short or however real, is something you should avoid.
- You should hide your powerful feelings in food rather than learn the appropriate—and healthier—response, which is to allow yourself to feel.
- In short, rather than feel your feelings, eat them.

"Have a cookie and everything will be all right" was the message this little girl's father silently gave his daughter. But instead of giving her food he could have hugged her and smoothed her hair. Eventually the pain would have eased and she would have stopped crying. Instead, at six months old she had already learned to "eat" her feelings instead of feeling them. And just as swiftly the chemical "hook" was in place, those sparks of physiological cravings created by the blast of sugar—staying ignited long after this particular incident was over.

Sound familiar?

A PROGRAM THAT WORKS

For the past eighteen years I have done absolutely nothing to promote myself or my diet program. I have not had a publicist. I have not sought out magazine writers or radio personalities. Yes, I have lectured to local groups who have asked, and responded to the magazines in which I have been quoted. But that is it. Yet in my private practice on Long Island and in Manhattan I see sixty-five to eighty-five clients every week—all of them from unsolicited referrals, from clients' word of mouth, or from doctors, therapists, and other health-related professionals. I have thousands of patients who come see me or phone me long-distance, from all walks of life, from all over the country.

Why did this happen?

Because what I offer works. My clients love my program and are very vocal about telling me. I cannot count how many people have told me that they do not know how they existed before, that I have saved their lives or changed their lives, or that they just wanted to say thank you, thank you, thank you. I cannot count how many kisses I've had or hugs of joy.

A large percentage of my clients are high-profile personalities. I have many CEOs of Fortune 500 companies, actors, socialites, sports figures, and people who could live next door.

Until now I have been too busy to actually write a book about my diet plan, but my clients have asked me so many times to put my thoughts on paper that I can no longer ignore their pleas. If I can help them, I know I can help you, too.

THE REVOLUTIONARY 5-DAY MIRACLE DIET

In a nutshell the 5-Day Miracle Diet is based on controlling the physiological urges that cause you to go off diets, cheat on diets, and not stay within the goal weights you have set up.

It is not difficult. It is easy to follow. It is portable and can go with you when you travel, when you entertain, when you eat in a restaurant or at someone's house. It will get you through holidays, weddings, bar mitzvahs, and even the vicissitudes of life that make you want to grab a pint of politically incorrect ice cream and never let go.

It's all here, within the pages of this book. And step by step I'll be with you, offering advice, information, insight, and even a laugh or two.

You will find out how your body works, why blood-sugar levels are so critical, and why my diet is so different from anything else you've ever tried. You will also learn how to deal with the psychological ramifications of your diet program—and how the *fathead* can adjust to you, your needs, and your desires.

You will even discover how to fit regular exercise into your busy routine—as well as some easy, delicious "cooking with vegetables" hints and recipes you and your whole family will enjoy.

Imagine. No more cravings. No more mood swings. No more need for naps in the middle of the day. Instead the 5-Day Miracle Diet will give you:

- Robust health
- Steady weight loss that's maintained over the long haul
- Energy that just won't quit
- An incredible sense of well-being

As Ellie recently said to me, "I've been waiting my whole life for this. I can't believe how good I feel."

Now you don't have to come to my office. You don't have to go any farther than the next page of this book. It's your turn and I'm here to help. Whether you're fifty or fifteen, an older woman or a younger man, a businessperson or a homebody, on a budget or on an expense account, this diet will work for you.

It might seem like a miracle, but it's not.

It's a proven fact.

Let's begin. . . .

ADELE'S FORMULA FOR SUCCESS

Adherence to program = No physiological cravings + No psychological deprivation = Reasonable eating = *SUCCESS!*

CHAPTER 1

Debunking the Myths

*If I had known about this in high school,
who knows? I could have been a rocket
scientist.*
    —Lisa, a thirty-two-year-old teacher

While I was studying metabolic rates, biochemical reactions, and food content for my master's degree, I was also investigating diets on my own—for a very good reason. As you already know, the "Green genes" were always ready to pounce and make me fat. Either I was twenty or thirty pounds overweight or looking to lose only five more pounds. Even when I was thin, it was a struggle to stay there. In my quest for the perfect diet, a program that would keep weight off for good, I came across many diet "icons" that turned out to be completely false—and even detrimental to sound weight loss.

Before we go on to the 5-Day Miracle Diet, let's test your diet savvy and take a look at some of the diet myths that refuse to, well, die.

TEST YOUR DIET SAVVY

Spend a few moments to take this quiz—and see what you know about diets and food. What you learn will help you separate the good from the bad, the healthful from the dangerous, the diets you've already tried from the one you're about to begin. You might even find a surprise or two!

TRUE OR FALSE

1. *You have to deprive yourself to lose weight.*
2. *Motivation is the key to success for any diet.*
3. *If indulge you must, go for the "lite"!*
4. *Expect plateaus on any diet.*
5. *Think food pyramid if you want to lose weight healthfully.*
6. *Bananas, yogurt, bagels—all these are great diet foods.*
7. *The first few pounds you lose don't count. It's only water weight.*
8. *You should take advantage of the diet foods that stock your grocery shelves.*

Did you agree with any of these statements? Believe it or not, every single one of these "diet principles" is *false*. Let's go over each one of these diet myths now and see why.

Die-hard Diet Myth 1: You Have to Deprive Yourself to Lose Weight

We all know this one. In other guises it's called the "cottage cheese and lettuce club," the "water and dry-fish approach," and of course the ever-popular "a shake for breakfast, a shake for lunch, and a sensible meal for dinner."

As one comedian put it, what is sensible? After drinking those liquid shakes for an entire day, a sensible meal is anything you can order and consume in five minutes or less, the more gooey, sugary, and fatty the better.

Even though countless diet programs have said you can have your cake and eat it, too, in your heart of hearts, you have that "nibbling" doubt: For a diet to really work, you have to sacrifice.

I know. I bought into this myth for a long time myself.

And the fact is that on every other diet, deprivation is involved. Motivation can only take you so far. Eventually you're going to grab for that extra piece of cake, that box of cookies, that cheeseburger and fries.

But not on the 5-Day Miracle Diet. My program goes right to the source: the biology of our cravings, or, in other words, the chemical and hormonal imbalances that make us feel deprived and make other diets fail. You will learn to control both the physical and the emotional deprivations that are inescapable in every other diet. You will learn that there are no food "villains." And as you will see, I even *insist* that you eat something you absolutely adore once or twice a week!

Even in today's health-savvy times, more than half of the American diet comes from "empty" calories: sugar, alcohol, and fat.

Die-hard Diet Myth 2: Motivation Is the Key to Success for Any Diet

This myth is very much linked to the "deprivation" lie—only it goes deeper. Not only does it mean you must fight the feelings of "deprivation" every diet inflicts, but, when your white-knuckled mode says "enough!" you also get to feel guilt:

"I failed—again."

"I'm just not strong enough."

"Let's face it. I just can't lose weight."

Sound familiar? We've all said these things—including me—at one time or another in our lives. But the fact is that motivation, inspiration, and willpower will take you only so far. It's not only a question of mind over matter. We're talking about a physical phenomenon here, a physical reaction in your body that *demands* food—now. How can anyone fight a force as powerful as that?

In short, motivation is only one small factor in a successful diet program. Once I've shown you how to control your body chemistry, you will no longer have those physiological cravings that make anyone's motivation go out the window. You will glide through your days, healthy and energetic, without giving what you're *not* eating a second thought.

Die-hard Diet Myth 3: If Indulge You Must, Go for the "Lite"!

One of my clients, Bonnee, followed my program explicitly. She did everything right—except for one thing. When I told her she could have salad dressing, she headed for the "no-fat" ones. When it came to her bread selections, she'd go for whole wheat—"lite" whole wheat, that is. When she chose her weekly food favorite, she'd always pick nonfat frozen yogurt, "lite" brownies, or no-fat Fig Newtons.

After a few weeks of "lite" eating, the weight she'd lost began to creep back on. Worse, her food cravings were as bad as they were before she started my program.

When I discovered what Bonnee had been doing, I knew exactly what the problem was: She was eating too much "lite" food—and enjoying it less.

There's a reason why the familiar diet cookies, yogurts, and ice-cream products are displayed so prominently in our supermarkets today. They sell. According to a recent *Newsweek* article, SnackWell's cookies outsold Oreos, Lorna Doones, and Chips Ahoy! in 1994. People are buying into this myth with a vengeance. If something is low-fat, it has to be good—and low in calories, too.

Unfortunately many people, like Bonnee, are discovering that low-fat can be a sham. The fact is that fat tastes good. We like it in our cookies, our cakes, our sauces, our Caesar salads. If that fat is taken away, something has to replace it to satisfy our taste buds. That "something" is usually sugar. Look at the no-fat salad dressings on your supermarket shelves. Chances are sugar (or one of its derivatives, such as maltose, sucrose, fructose, or corn syrup) has taken the place of fat. And that sugar helps perpetuate a chemical imbalance in our bodies, creating cravings and a nosedive into that not-so-low-in-calories-anymore carton of low-fat cake.

A small amount of fat is a necessary part of my program. You *need* a certain amount of fat. Your body cannot manufacture enough of the essential fatty acids it needs for good health, proper digestion, strong nails, and glowing skin. And because your food cravings will disappear on my program within a week, you won't overeat fat. Indeed, once or twice a week on my program you will walk right past that "low-fat" display in the supermarket and head out the door for the French bistro down the block, where perhaps you'll order a warm baguette and cheese, or a scrumptious pastry—because you can!

▲ ▲ ▲ ▲ ▲ ▲ ▲ ▲ ▲

ARE YOU FAT-PHOBIC?

Take too much of a good thing and you can develop a phobia. Watching your fat is a healthy
thing to do, but eliminating it from your diet, ob-
sessing about it, and spending your life reading
labels is not. Take this quiz and see if you are
"fat-phobic":

   You always look for the word *lite* on breads,
      cheeses, and spreads.
   You constantly ask your trainer or physician to
      measure your body fat.
   You won't eat grilled vegetables in a restaurant
      because they have a slight touch of oil.
   Even when you told the waiter "no oil," you
      don't believe there's none on your plate
      when your entrée is in front of you.
   You haven't tasted a "real" cookie in over six
      months.
   If a restaurant doesn't have skim milk, you'll
      forgo the coffee . . .
      . . . and you won't even entertain the
      thought of cappuccino (which, incidentally,
      only has thirty calories).
   You always eat fish broiled and dry—even
      though you hate it.

   If you answered yes to any of these questions,
you might have to reexamine your relationship
with fat.

▼ ▼ ▼ ▼ ▼ ▼ ▼ ▼ ▼

Die-hard Diet Myth 4: Expect Plateaus on Any Diet

It was always the same. Melissa would go on a diet, lose
two or three pounds consistently every week, and then, as
if a giant sign popped up proclaiming "No More," the
weight loss would suddenly stop. The diet specialists she
went to all said the same thing:

"You've hit a plateau. Keep going. The weight will start to come off again."

"Reduce your calories and you'll start to lose." (Even though Melissa was already on a meager 1,100-calorie-a-day diet!)

"Exercise more. You'll see the weight drop." (Even though Melissa was already exercising every day for one hour on her treadmill!)

Unfortunately the "plateau" eroded Melissa's motivation, which, after several weeks, was already becoming increasingly "white-knuckled." She felt disgusted and frustrated. She didn't know how to lose any more weight. She promptly went off her diet—again.

The "diet plateau" has long been a mystery, a magical word for those times when weight doesn't come off. The reality is that there are no such things as "plateaus." If you are following my program of food and exercise, you will not have any plateaus. If your body has good chemistry, the weight will continue to drop off, slowly and consistently.

There are of course weight fluctuations, times when your weight changes by a pound or two or even three. But this is to be expected. Muscle weighs more than fat, and when you begin to exercise (a crucial component of my program), you might experience a minor weight gain. Further, it takes your body a few weeks to "catch up" to your new, healthier lifestyle.

But fluctuations are not plateaus. And in the long run (no pun intended), the diet you are eating and the exercise you are doing will "jump-start" your metabolism. You'll know when to exercise more to burn more calories—and when to take a time-out because you're losing weight too fast.

I don't believe in the word *plateau*. It doesn't exist in the 5-Day Miracle Diet world. It is a place without such walls, such obstacles.

When Melissa reached a place where she wasn't losing weight for several weeks on my program, we examined what she'd been eating. Sure enough, she'd gone out to eat Japanese food three times, eating low-calorie but high-sodium foods—which caused water retention. Add the fact that work prevented her from going to the gym four times and you don't have to be P. D. James to solve this "Mystery of the Plateau." A little examining, a little analyzing, a little planning—such as getting back to the gym and staying away from salty foods—and Melissa soon began to lose weight again.

Again, there are no such things as "plateaus" when you're on the 5-Day Miracle Diet. If you're not losing weight for a few weeks in a row, there will always be a reason you can identify—not some mysterious, magical "plateau." *You're* in charge on my program. You'll know what to do. That's a promise.

Die-hard Diet Myth 5: Think Food Pyramid If You Want to Lose Weight Healthfully

From cereal boxes to weight-loss classes, the carbo-heavy food pyramid is all the news. According to the American Heart Association, the American Dietetics Association, and the American Diabetes Association, our daily intake of food should consist of 60 percent carbohydrates. Next in line are fruits and vegetables, then protein, milk products, and a small 20 to 30 percent of fats at the very top.

All well and good. In theory this does make for healthy eating. But these pyramids do not tell you what *kinds* of carbohydrates, vegetables, and fruits to eat. And if you happen to be insulin resistant or a carbohydrate addict, the food pyramid can actually be hazardous to your health. A study at Stanford University School of Medicine found that a high-carbohydrate diet can raise triglyceride levels and lower "good" or HDL cholesterol in people who are insulin resistant. These people usually have high blood pressure and, as they age, develop diabetes. Dr. George Raven of Stanford University calls this Syndrome X, a condition that puts you at great risk for heart disease.

If you reduce the amount of insulin your body produces, you also reduce its production of eicosanoids, the "overseeing" hormones that "tell" the body to create insulin in the first place. I'll be discussing the role of insulin in the 5-Day Miracle Diet in the next chapter (and carbohydrate addiction later on), but suffice it to say that today's food pyramid is perfectly fine, but, like the ancient ones in the pharaohs' time, certain elements within that pyramid make it easy to rob and plunder.

Note the food pyramid below. The food groups represented are healthful and the amounts are correct. But look closely at the pictures within each group:

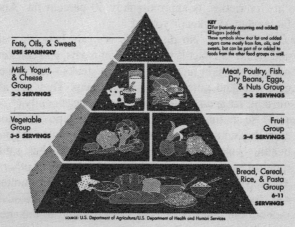

KEY
☐ Fat (naturally occurring and added)
☑ Sugars (added)
These symbols show that fat and added sugars come mostly from fats, oils, and sweets, but can be part of or added to foods from the other food groups as well.

Fats, Oils, & Sweets
USE SPARINGLY

Milk, Yogurt, & Cheese Group
2-3 SERVINGS

Meat, Poultry, Fish, Dry Beans, Eggs, & Nuts Group
2-3 SERVINGS

Vegetable Group
3-5 SERVINGS

Fruit Group
2-4 SERVINGS

Bread, Cereal, Rice, & Pasta Group
6-11 SERVINGS

SOURCE: U.S. Department of Agriculture/U.S. Department of Health and Human Services

Carbohydrates: A croissant is almost 80 percent fat. And the white-flour rolls and breadsticks will keep you in low blood sugar—and craving more.

Vegetables: Peas, corn, and acorn squash are starchy. They, too, can keep you in low blood sugar. People overload on these particular veggies, ignoring others that also contain nutrients and fiber—with less calories and more blood sugar balance capability.

Fruits: Sure, bananas, pineapples, and melons taste great—and they are chock-full of vitamins. But they are also chock-full of natural sugar, which can keep your blood sugar imbalanced and your cravings continuous. There are better choices within the fruit group for losing weight and keeping cravings at bay.

Dairy Products: Calcium can be found in other items besides milk and yogurt. The lactose in milk can promote an overproduction of insulin—and, yes, keep blood-sugar levels low. Yogurt is very easily assimilated because it is almost digestible without the body contributing much to the process. In addition cheese, even "lite" varieties, is approximately 60 percent fat. And fat, as they say, keeps you fat.

Protein Products: No distinction is made between fish and steak. The fact is that fish, lean meats, and chicken without the skin have less fat than steaks—and fewer calories. And nuts? Forget about them. They are almost all fat and should be used only occasionally.

Fats: "Use sparingly" is one thing, but the type of fat you spread or cook with can also make a difference in your health. Unsaturated fats are *always* better than saturated ones. And some of these are better than others. To keep "bad" cholesterol (LDL) low, polyunsaturated oils, such as canola and safflower, are best. Olive oil, a monounsaturated fat, has also been found to enhance "good" cholesterol (HDL) levels.

On my program the food pyramid is definitely in place, but you will find that the specific foods you'll be eating at specific times during the day will give you more energy, help you lose weight, and help you feel better than you ever have in your life. Instead of grabbing the "low-end" sugary, fatty foods your body is making you crave, you'll reach for the "high-end," high-quality foods that will make you feel, well, like a queen—or king—of the Nile.

FATTY ISSUES

Unsaturated fats keep cholesterol at bay better than those ubiquitous saturated fats. But within the unsaturated-fat category, there are mono-unsaturated fats, which laboratory studies have found lower only "bad" LDL cholesterol, and polyunsaturated fats, which lower both "bad" LDL and "good" HDL cholesterol. Here's a sampling:

Saturated Fats	Monounsaturated	Polyunsaturated
Butter	Olive oil	Safflower oil
Animal fat	Canola oil	Corn oil
Shortening	Peanut oil	Soybean oil
Palm oil		Sunflower oil
Coconut oil		Margarine
		(made with liquid
		vegetable oil)

Die-hard Diet Myth 6: Bananas, Yogurt, Bagels— All These Are Great Diet Foods

How many of us have started diets that included a low-fat yogurt for a snack? Or a plain bagel for breakfast? And don't forget that ever-important, easy-to-eat banana— whenever the mood hits.

And while we're at it, how many diets have you been on where you didn't start to crave other foods within a few weeks? What about gaining and losing that same ten pounds over and over again?

Most likely you've blamed yourself, your weak will, your lack of motivation, when in actuality most of the reasons stem from those very same "diet" foods that are purportedly so good for you.

Bagels, yogurt, bananas, and other foods you'll be reading about are all absorbed by the body very quickly. They create a sudden, immediate hormonal rush into your bloodstream. They cause a chemical imbalance that leads to low blood sugar.

And the low blood sugar triggers a craving for more . . . bagels, yogurt, and, yes, bananas.

My diet is different. It's all about achieving and maintaining good blood sugar—and that means thinking about and being affected by food in a totally different way.

YES, WE HAVE NO BANANAS

When the first doctor gave his first patient the suggestion to eat a banana for extra potassium, he had no idea the precedent he was setting.

Sure, bananas are easy to eat. People like them. They will eat them. And it's true that they are high in potassium.

But there are a lot of other foods that are also chock-full of potassium and are better for you, including broccoli, potatoes, grapefruit, and many other vegetables and fruits.

Die-hard Diet Myth 7: The First Few Pounds You Lose Don't Count—It's Only Water Weight

When Alex got on the scale after a week on my program, he'd lost five pounds. He should have been elated. Instead he shrugged his shoulders. "Big deal," he said. "It's only water."

I don't know about you, but to me, weight loss is weight loss. Five pounds *off* your body weight is better than *on*—and saying "It's only water" is negative thinking and ultimately self-defeating.

When fat is broken down in your system, it is converted into liquid. One ounce of fat equals four and a half ounces of fluid. The elimination of that liquid is a sign that fat is dissolving. The liquid itself? Water. Sounds like real weight loss to me!

Die-hard Diet Myth 8: You Should Take Advantage of the Diet Foods That Stock Your Grocery Shelves

Unfortunately those frozen boxes with tantalizing pictures of "diet" éclairs, ice-cream bars, and fettucine Alfredo might look luscious, but they are not going to help your diet. As with many of the foods we've already exposed, these too are dangerous to your blood-sugar health. Studies have found that artificial sweeteners can trigger the need for a sugar "hit." Whether it is fructose, sucrose, or NutraSweet, sugar substances and sugar substitutes can create blood-sugar imbalances. Fructose, supposedly a "purer" form of sugar because it is found in fruits and vegetables, might be better than a teaspoon of the white refined variety, but it too can create havoc.

Unfortunately sugar—whether artificial sweetener or "the real thing"—is rarely found without another carbohydrate, whether it be fruit, vegetable, or an ice-milk pop. And, further, it is seldom consumed without a "hit" and a desire for more. Rather than help you lose weight, diet products ultimately encourage you to eat more!

▲   ▲   ▲   ▲   ▲   ▲   ▲   ▲   ▲

STOP AND SMELL THE "OSES"

I tell my clients to watch for the "oses," those
sugars that are listed on packages that aren't
spelled s-u-g-a-r. Some of the "oses" include:

- Maltose   • Fructose
- Sucrose   • Dextrose

▼   ▼   ▼   ▼   ▼   ▼   ▼   ▼   ▼

These are only a few of the diet myths I've encountered in my journey toward the "perfect diet"—the 5-Day
Miracle Diet. As you read on, you'll learn more things
about diets, foods, psychological saboteurs, and body
chemistry that just might astound you.

And they will definitely help you lose weight!

CHAPTER 2

The Chemistry Connection

I have been trying to lose weight for more years than I care to remember. This is the first time that a weight-loss program has worked, and worked better than I could have ever expected.
—A thirty-nine-year-old playwright

Every time I sit down with a new client, I think about Danny. He was a tall, strapping man with a joie de vivre about him. He loved his family, his work, his leisure time—and his food. Danny loved to eat, and eat he did, until he was forty pounds overweight.

When I explained the simple formula behind my diet, he didn't believe me. He shook his head. "That's it? Chemistry?"

"That's it," I told him. "Stabilizing blood-sugar levels."

Danny was skeptical. "You mean if I eat the way you're telling me, I'll lose my cravings for fattening food in five days?"

"Yes. Absolutely yes."

Danny was not atypical in his reaction. Most of my clients are skeptical at first. They can't believe how simple the solution is—or that the reason they've not lost weight is largely a physical one.

What made Danny different from my other clients was the way he handled the program. He lost some weight, but it was always a struggle. Week after week he came in to my office, bigger than life, ready to tell me about the scrumptious bagel and gravlax he had on Sunday, the charbroiled filet mignon Saturday night, the blue cheese dressing, and the crème brûlée for dessert.

I'd look right at him. "Why, Danny?" I would ask. "Why aren't you following the program?"

Danny always had the same answer: "The devil made me do it."

Although Danny was kidding, in actuality there really is a "devil" that makes you eat. It's called low blood sugar, and it's the major reason you haven't had success on any other diet before.

THE BAD-BLOOD-SUGAR-BLUES QUIZ

Low blood sugar, or as I call it, "bad" blood sugar, is much more common than you might think. Do you . . .

1. Have a plain bagel for breakfast?
2. Wait to eat breakfast until you get to work?
3. Have frozen yogurt for lunch or dinner because you think it is a good diet meal?
4. Have cereals that list sugar as an ingredient?
5. Feel that raisins are a necessary addition to your cereal?
6. Have pasta for lunch because you feel it's a healthy, low-fat food?
7. Eat peanut butter that contains sugar?
8. Drink juice as part of your morning routine?
9. Tend to combine breakfast and lunch into one meal called "brunch" on weekends?
10. Tend to eat those lo-cal, low-fat diet hard candies, thinking they are okay?
11. Often have lunchtime meetings that don't include food?
12. Overeat at lunch, then skip dinner?

13. Feel diet cookies or desserts are a "have to have" daily ritual?
14. Chew gum as if it's an essential food?
15. Drink lots of diet sodas and other diet drinks?
16. Use diet sweeteners?
17. Tend to "push" to the next town when on a trip instead of stopping for lunch at a reasonable hour?
18. Wait to have breakfast until you board a plane?
19. Not particularly want to go out anywhere?
20. Yawn a lot around three to four in the afternoon?
21. Find you can't stay focused at work?
22. Feel sleepy most of the time?
23. Frequently feel dizzy and light-headed?
24. Feel tired all the time?
25. Like to sleep in on your days off?
26. Get heart palpitations?
27. Get migraine headaches so much, they are "ingrained" in you?
28. Sometimes feel as if you can't catch your breath?
29. Feel sad without knowing why?
30. Believe you're moderately depressed?
31. Have little energy?
32. Have little desire to meet new people?
33. Find sex uninteresting?
34. Crave starches—any kind of bread, pasta, or cake?
35. Sometimes wake up in the middle of the night to eat something sweet?
36. Need to drink coffee all the time?
37. Have to have at least two drinks at dinner?
38. Get really irritable?
39. Always feel nervous?
40. Have insomnia?
41. Fly off the handle for no reason?
42. Always feel hungry?
43. Have weight problems?

44. Have dull-looking skin?
45. Experience mood swings, where one minute you are elated, the next, down in the dumps?
46. Look pale and washed out?
47. Have problems sitting still?
48. Remember *not* feeling depressed?
49. Adore food so much, you think about it all the time?
50. Hate food so much, you think about it all the time?

If more than five of these questions ring true for you, you could very well be in bad blood sugar—and it's seriously affecting the quality of your life.

Think about it. Bad blood sugar creates a tired feeling and excessive yawning in the middle of the afternoon, a poor night's sleep, forgetfulness, lethargy, crankiness, mood swings, heart palpitations, depression, dizziness, and a lack of energy. None of these conditions exactly help you live up to your full potential—but don't despair. You're not alone.

When *anyone* is in bad blood sugar, he or she will crave that cookie, that chocolate bar, even that blueberry yogurt with granola. You are quite simply out of control. How can you fight a force as powerful as this?

GLUCOSE: FOOD OF THE GODS

Glucose is *the* food of your body. It feeds your heart, muscles, and internal organs. Glucose is the only food your brain uses as fuel—and it cannot be stored for future use. The glucose your brain "eats" every day enhances brain activity, energy levels, and emotions. Bad blood sugar doesn't enhance brain activity; it alters it the minute you get into a bad-blood-sugar state from eating the wrong things. It can make you spacey, forgetful, anxious, depressed, unable to concentrate, and it can even stifle your creativity!

Once we've eaten, the foods we've ingested are broken down in our liver, which sits above our stomach. The carbohydrates, vegetables, fruits, and processed foods we'd first swallowed are separated into various components, including toxic materials and indigestible matter, which are eliminated via the intestines, and glucose, or blood sugar. This all-important glucose has to travel throughout our body to feed hungry cells.

But glucose needs additional help to be broken down to its "body fuel" state. And it also needs help to make the journey fast and smooth. And that's where insulin and glucagon come in.

THE CHEMISTRY CONNECTION:
HOW YOUR BODY WORKS

When you consume food, you work your mouth and jaw. This in turn stimulates the pituitary gland, a small pealike gland in the brain that sits at the point where your jaws meet your cheekbones. Just to make sure it's sufficiently stimulated, your pituitary gland also gets a message from the busily working liver via the brain: Stimulate the pancreas, which happens to conveniently sit below the stomach. Your pancreas dutifully manufactures two hormones that travel to the liver. One is glucagon, a hormone that joins the mix in the liver to break down the sugars even further. Ultimately glucagon breaks down sugar to its primal state: glucose. Now the body can "eat."

The other hormone your pancreas secretes is insulin, which moves the now-pure glucose out of the liver into the bloodstream and ultimately into the body's cells for energy.

When glucose levels traveling around your bloodstream are balanced and stable, you experience a state of "good blood sugar." You feel more energetic, more productive, and more focused.

However, if too little glucose is made available to your cells, a state of low blood sugar is created. Your body experiences uncontrollable cravings for certain foods at certain times—simultaneously sending the brain messages of longing for its food, glucose, which is found in carbohydrates such as alcohol, sugar, fruit, starches, and, to a much lesser degree, vegetables.

In this way low blood sugar becomes your body's "ventriloquist," commanding you to eat the food it needs to replenish its glucose levels—fast. In other words low blood sugar controls the body and tells it what to do, what to eat, and what to ask for in the way of food. In a state of low blood sugar, the glucagon in your body is diminished. When it is not replenished at the right time, havoc reigns.

"Give me glucose!" the brain cries.

And the body complies—with a starchy, sugary carboladen "hit" people particularly adore, the alcohol, chocolate, candy, ice cream, cake, and cookies that, when disassembled in the liver, contain an abundant amount of . . . glucose.

Danny's "devil made me do it" is not so far off the mark.

The brain requires 400 calories of glucose every day, and if it's not continuously "fed," you will die within minutes.

THE PHYSIOLOGY OF A CRAVING

Unfortunately the simple carbohydrates, such as the ubiquitous alcohol, chocolate, candy, ice cream, cake, and cookies, are so easily dismantled that the glucose is rapidly released and "rushed" into your bloodstream, creating an alarmist state in your body. Too much circulating glucose causes your body to enter an imbalanced state. "Danger," your brain now seems to say. "Glucose overload. Poison."

Your pancreas, suddenly faced with an immense job, can only direct itself to one goal: Get rid of the glucose *immediately* by producing large amounts of insulin. The insulin the pancreas produces zooms in, working so hard, so fast, and so diligently that the rug is literally pulled out from underfoot and you are left in a state of low blood sugar.

The result? A craving. Your body wants something. It doesn't know it needs a more balanced, homeostatic state. It just knows it wants something . . . such as another chocolate bar.

If you are like so many other "professional" dieters, you are always promising to *never* eat another piece of chocolate again, when, twenty-five to forty-five minutes later, the craving, like a sledgehammer, "hits" you once more. You're still not finished. The easily absorbed sugary carbs are converted and gobbled up so fast that your blood sugar drops very low and your body needs to eat again. It starts crying "Feed me," seducing the brain to respond quickly.

"Give me milk chocolate with peanuts," your brain demands. And unfortunately, no matter how much willpower you might have, eventually you will succumb.

There is simply no way you can resist your body's physiological needs—unless you begin to orchestrate your own chemistry.

Chemistry stabilization is made more difficult by the

fact that the foods that create blood-sugar swings are not always as obvious as a chocolate bar. Items such as yogurt, bagels, oranges, bananas, and yes, even pasta can create havoc in your system. They are all highly glycemic; they contain simple carbohydrates and are too quickly converted into glucose.

You do not have to be hypoglycemic to have low, or, as I describe it to my clients, bad blood sugar. The impact of glucose is felt by everyone. In fact most people live in bad blood sugar. The way they eat, the types of food they eat, and the times they eat cause erratic emotion, behavior, and energy levels that are typical of bad blood sugar.

ADRENALINE: THE ICING ON THE GLYCEMIC CAKE

Bad blood sugar also affects the way your body metabolizes food. The alarmist state that occurs when you are in bad blood sugar also stimulates the adrenal glands, which are located near the kidneys, into manufacturing yet another hormone—adrenaline. This adrenaline is the chemical that gives us that quick shot of energy. It is your body's literal cry for help.

The brain complies and sends out its own message, one as old as the hills, as old as the days when prehistoric peoples hunted and fought for their survival.

"Give me energy!" the brain says, and the adrenal glands comply.

"Fight or flight!" is the adrenaline's answer. In prehistoric cultures adrenaline was a prayer come true. The quick dash of energy would help people run away from a woolly mammoth—or give them the strength to kill it. Metabolism would rise, calories would burn, and as soon as the danger was over, their bodies would go back to normal stasis.

The adrenal glands also worked hand in hand with the pituitary gland in those long-ago days. Tribes often went without food; they died of starvation. To help people conserve their energy, the brain issued another comandment: "Go slow. Conserve fuel." Thus less food (glucose) was burned for energy; metabolism was slowed.

Our bodies don't realize we're about to enter the twenty-first century. When we feel stress on the job, at home, or in the middle of the night, the adrenal glands start working. The heart starts pumping; we are alert, full of hyperenergy. Unfortunately the fight-or-flight message doesn't find relief. There's no immediate danger to run away from, no mammoth to kill. We're left in an imbalanced, stressed-out state. The free-floating adrenaline that's responsible for this alarmist, heightened state joins forces with the excess insulin that's already in place from our bad-blood-sugar mode, and a megapowerful craving is created.

Add a low-calorie, low-blood-sugar, restrictive diet to this brew and your body gets *really* confused. Now your brain thinks it needs to conserve energy; it thinks "starvation mode." It doesn't know that you've spurned breakfast and lunch out of choice, because you want to lose weight. After all, in long-ago days, food was catch as catch can. Obesity didn't exist. Suddenly you find yourself thinking about food, dreaming about food. Ultimately the diet goes out the window. And, because your metabolism has slowed, it doesn't take long for you to gain back your weight—and then some. It makes sense that 97 percent of the people who go on diets regain their weight within two years!

And it all started with that first cookie or lollipop or candy bar you found so delicious so many years ago.

CONTROLLING THE FOOD
SENSUALIST IN ALL OF US

There is only one way to halt this powerful force: by stabilizing your blood-sugar level. Creating a state of *good* blood sugar by eating a combination of different foods and textures at specific times during the day—which will get rid of the highs, throw away the lows, and give you balanced, more focused energy the whole day through.

THE CHINESE NOODLE STORY

When a new client comes in, I usually begin our session with a story about myself.

I don't particularly love Chinese noodles. They're all right. I like them, but there are many other things I'd rather eat. When I was younger (remember those "Green genes?"), I'd start to eat the noodles before ordering my food, dipping them into the duck sauce and the hot mustard without thinking.

Today, when I'm in bad blood sugar, they still talk to me. They croon. They whisper passionately and I can't help myself. Before I know it, I've dipped. It's an unconscious act. And if an unfortunate waiter happens to come by to take them away, I'd actually think about pushing his or her hand away!

So-so blood sugar is a little better. I *know* I shouldn't eat the noodles; I'm still in control. But they are tempting. They are staring at me. In situations like this I'll put a few on my plate and then ask the waiter to take the rest away—immediately!

But when I'm in good blood sugar, *I don't even notice*

them. The noodles could be calling out my name and waving their crunchy, tasty arms—and I would not see or hear anything.

That's how powerful blood sugar is—and how empowering my program can be.

▬ ▬ ▬ ▬ ▬ ▬ ▬ ▬ ▬

Think of cellulite as metabolic sludge. It's fat, true, but a specialized fat, one that comes from a metabolically "dirty" diet—as opposed to the metabolically clean 5-Day Miracle Diet. If you don't eat right, waste products cause fat to be stored under the skin, creating that "orange-peel-y" look. The worse you eat, the more fat and sugar, the more cellulite you'll have.

Men get cellulite, too. It just so happens that their skin is thicker, so it doesn't show.

Who says life is fair?

▬ ▬ ▬ ▬ ▬ ▬ ▬ ▬ ▬

THE 5-DAY MIRACLE DIET: NO MORE CRAVINGS

My plan is simple—and it works. It regulates your blood sugar by using specific times you must eat, specific types of food you must eat, and specific combinations of foods you must eat.

Eating at specific times helps restore blood-sugar balance. By properly spacing out your foods, the enzymes that break down your food in your digestive system have a "routine." They know when to rest—and when to work.

Eating specific foods—and specific combinations—helps maintain the proper balance of insulin and glucagon the pancreas produces. This in turn makes for a well-tuned body.

My diet is also metabolically clean. It gears and primes your system for the threefold process of eating:

ingest, digest (break down), and eliminate. The foods you eat not only satisfy your cells, but they act as "scrubbing brushes," cleaning out your cells and helping with elimination—as opposed to foods that create water retention because they are *not* efficient metabolically. These include, yes, those sugary, salty, carbo-and-fat-laden foods our body craves when in a state of bad blood sugar.

My program is specifically designed to work with the body—not against it. In short, if you follow my diet plan, you will be in good blood sugar, which means that the ups and downs of life, those rejections and those anxieties, those celebrations and those temptations, will not have you reaching into the freezer. You will pick and choose what you want to eat. You will know how to be prepared. You will enjoy life even more because you are no longer controlled by the subtle ventriloquist called low blood sugar.

Are you ready to feel better than you ever have?

Are you ready to feel absolutely fabulous?

Without any further ado, let's go on to the actual 5-Day Miracle Diet itself. . . .

FOOD FOR THOUGHT

The 5-Day Miracle Diet is not about *never* eating certain things ever again. It's learning how to live harmoniously with your food.

CHAPTER 3

The 5-Day Miracle Diet: The Last Diet You Will Ever Need!

I feel like you saved my life.
—A twenty-eight-year-old sales manager

Listen:

"Vegetables in the morning? Forget about it!"

"I can't live without my bagel!"

"I need to eat after dinner. I have to have that late-night snack."

"If I don't eat my banana, where do I get my potassium?"

"No orange juice? I've been drinking it in the morning all my life."

These sentences are not lines of dialogue from a new play. They are all real comments made by my clients when they first came to see me.

The diet you are about to discover is so revolutionary, so different, that you, too, might say something similar, think something similar, or simply want to toss the book away.

Don't.

I guarantee that in five days, if you follow the program, you will feel completely different about the foods you eat. You will also discover that nothing is taken away from you—except weight and that sluggish feeling. My program is based on a sound, reasonable philosophy. And if you are in good blood sugar, you will not only

41

have learned to eat reasonably well, you will *want* to eat reasonably well.

Take away low blood sugar and you remove the body's ventriloquist, the seductive voice with the bad ideas. You will feel better than you ever have in your life.

Now that you know what good blood sugar is, here are the nuts and bolts to get you there. It's not a magic yellow brick road. It's not hocus-pocus nonsense. It's a reasonable diet using reasonable amounts of food at reasonable times of day.

The results will astound you.

Period.

End of speech.

Let's go on to the 5-Day Miracle Diet now.

THE LAST DIET YOU WILL EVER NEED—OR WANT

Army veterans jump out of bed when the bugle sounds. And so will you. But even they find it tough. When you wake, you are in low blood sugar. You haven't eaten in hours and your blood sugar has been dropping all night long (if, that is, you've been sleeping and not eating midnight snacks!). Your goal? Raise that bad blood sugar to a balanced, middle ground.

You have to do it promptly. Your blood sugar continues to drop until you eat. If you wait too long to eat, your blood sugar will become so low, it will be difficult to correct. Most likely this is the way you have been living your life until now—waiting until you're starving, until you're feeling weird and crazy ("I'm too tired to eat. . . . I'm in a rush. . . . I'll grab something later").

So the first thing you must do is eat—hungry or not. Call it food insurance, a "policy" that will protect you from overeating later in the day.

▲ ▲ ▲ ▲ ▲ ▲ ▲ ▲ ▲

THE GOLFER WHO ATE BREAKFAST

One of my clients, a golf aficionado, was out on the green at seven-thirty one balmy Saturday morning. He met his partner there, and as they were choosing clubs, my client opened up a bag and took out two rice cakes and two slices of turkey. He began to eat.

His partner looked at him incredulously. "You're eating *that* for breakfast? Are you crazy?"

My client nodded, completely calm. "What about you? What did you eat for breakfast?"

"A muffin and coffee" was the reply.

"A fatty, sugar-laden muffin? A jolt of caffeine?" My client shook his head. "And you call *me* crazy?"

♥ ♥ ♥ ♥ ♥ ♥ ♥ ♥ ♥

ADELE PUHN'S STEP 1:
EAT WITHIN ONE-HALF HOUR OF WAKING UP.

If you exercise first thing in the morning, you can stretch this time to forty-five minutes. Breakfast is fast and easy to prepare. It simply consists of a protein and a starch. (See the food choices starting on page 100.) A slice of bread and a dollop of unsweetened peanut butter. Or two rice cakes and ½ cup of no-fat cottage cheese sprinkled with cinnamon. Or a bowl of cereal with skim or 1% milk. (Cereal is not appropriate every day, however. Although nutritionally good for you, cereal doesn't supply as strong a "cushion" as say, six-grain bread and a slice of no-fat cheese. Biochemically, cereal doesn't supply the cushion your body needs to sustain a balanced blood-sugar level.)

The reason for these combinations is completely chemical: The enzymes in your digestive tract quickly release the sugar in the carbohydrates. The liver immediately breaks this sugar down into its pure "body food": glucose. Insulin swoops down and rushes this easily broken-down glucose to the hungry cells—giving you an immediate, quick, and necessary rush.

The protein is more slowly metabolized; it doesn't signal the alarm that makes the insulin and the other hormones dash in. They come into the liver quietly, efficiently, and calmly. The protein, along with other essential elements, builds up evenly and reliably, supporting and cushioning the fast and furious "good blood sugar" the starch created—and preventing the crash that always follows a rush. (Remember that eleven A.M. "feed me" tune, when the muffin or bagel you've eaten is a distant memory and your body begins pondering what you're going to eat for lunch. Lunch? Forget about it. I need to eat now!)

TUNA FOR BREAKFAST

Why not? Tuna, tofu, chicken, or turkey are all good protein choices. After all, we eat other strong-flavored foods such as bacon or sausage for breakfast—and they're not only meat products, they're also high in fat!

A case in point is Arthur, a client who recently started the 5-Day Miracle Diet. Prior to my program he ate a plain bagel for breakfast every morning at his desk. He felt great at ten, even virtuous for his "low-calorie" meal, but by eleven-thirty his thoughts were starting to wander during a board meeting. He felt sleepy and couldn't wait until lunch. The quick rush from the highly glycemic, too-easily-broken-down white-starch bagel had no "safety net." There was nowhere for the "high" to go but down. Like gravity's pull, his body's chemistry brought Arthur down to the sluggish, unfocused, tired state of bad blood sugar—which remained with him all day.

The simple breakfast you eat on my program, a protein and a starch, is guaranteed to keep your blood-sugar level balanced until the first snack.

The moral? You get a supply of good blood sugar—and it sticks.

And speaking of snacks . . .

ADELE PUHN'S STEP 2: ALWAYS EAT A "HARD CHEW" SNACK WITHIN TWO HOURS OF *STARTING* BREAKFAST. YOU CAN EAT THIS SNACK SOONER THAN TWO HOURS, BUT NEVER LATER.

"Hard chew" does not mean biting into a number-2 pencil. It is the opposite of "soft chew" and it is a phrase I created to denote specific snacks that help raise and maintain your blood-sugar levels. (See hard-chew snack choices on page 90.) A crisp stalk of celery converts into glucose slowly as it enters the bloodstream. You have to bite into it, chew it, and digest it.

A raw carrot is a hard chew; carrot juice is not. The complexity of a raw carrot's fibrous package makes it harder to break down. And the more difficult a food is to break down, the slower and more even its glucose release. Another example: An apple is a hard-chew package; it's better for you than a baked apple. A baked apple is better than applesauce. And applesauce is better than apple juice.

A hard chew is exactly that: a fruit or vegetable that's hard to chew. This steady chewing process provides a slow release of sugar from the food. This slow release, in turn, evens out the glucose distribution and keeps blood-sugar levels balanced.

THE 5-DAY MIRACLE DIET BULLETIN

Vegetable snacks are *always* hard chews. They don't have enough natural sugar to be "soft" and still carry the chemistry.

A hard chew also stimulates the pituitary gland, helping it to control blood sugar by keeping levels on an even keel. It can calmly and systematically help regulate the amount of insulin the pancreas produces.

So. You've eaten your first hard-chew snack. Your blood-sugar levels have risen—but not enough.

ADELE PUHN'S STEP 3: EAT A SECOND "HARD-CHEW" SNACK WITHIN TWO HOURS OF YOUR FIRST "HARD-CHEW" IF IT'S NOT YET LUNCHTIME— EVEN IF YOU EAT IT *RIGHT BEFORE* LUNCH.

Two hours later, after you have eaten your first snack—a hard chew such as an apple or a handful of string beans—you *must* eat another snack if you're not yet eating lunch. Since your blood-sugar levels are not yet stabilized, this snack has to be another hard chew.

This snack gets your good blood sugar over the finish line. It's vital that you eat your hard chew two hours later—even if it means eating a carrot in your car, on your way to your lunch date, or even in your office as you put on your coat!

The vegetable hard chews contain less sugar than their fruit counterparts. I recommend your first "hard chew" be a vegetable. Of course if you hate the idea of eating veggies in the morning, then a fruit hard chew will do.

LITTLE SCRUBBING BRUSHES

Vegetables scrub out your cells, while the fruit you eat eliminates that "scrub-out" from your body. Combined with eight or more glasses of water, you have the vehicle to move that eliminated "scrub-out" through your intestines. In this way you'll not only lose weight on my diet, *you will also look thinner.* The 5-Day Miracle Diet eliminates waste and makes you less likely to retain fluid. It's a metabolically clean diet.

ADELE PUHN'S STEP 4:
EAT LUNCH NO LATER THAN ONE P.M.

Remember, it's not how close together you eat the meals but *how far apart* that causes problems. I prefer that you eat lunch by one o'clock, but it depends on the time you regularly get up. If you're a night owl, the "lunch by one o'clock" rule can be adjusted. (See sample schedules, pages 54–56.) However, no matter when your wake-up call, even if you've nibbled your last cauliflower florette only five minutes ago, lunch should be on time.

Lunch includes protein and vegetables, either a large salad or a stir-fried or steamed dish. Bread is optional at lunch, unless you choose one of the vegetarian meals on page 83. If you are eating a vegetarian meal, you must substitute a starch for the animal protein—a starch other than bread or pasta. They are not as stabilizing as potatoes, beans, rice, or other grains. (See food choices starting on page 85.)

There are only two set rules concerning starchy carbohydrates on the 5-Day Miracle Diet:

1. *You cannot save bread for the evening meal,* because your metabolism is slower in the evening and calories eaten at night stay on the body.
2. *Never eat pasta at lunch—and limit pasta to only twice a week.* It's too glycemic, too easily broken down into simple sugars, just like your alcohol, bagels, yogurt, and cookies. Foods that are too glycemic create drowsiness and cravings.

Lunch should also include a small amount of hard-chew vegetables, not as much as you'd eat as snacks but just enough to "tie the bow on your stable blood-sugar package."

Congratulations! Your blood sugar is now stabilized. That's all it took. Now you simply have to keep in balanced blood sugar for the rest of the day.

ADELE PUHN'S STEP 5: EAT ONE OR TWO MORE SNACKS DURING THE AFTERNOON, SPACED NO FARTHER THAN THREE HOURS APART.

One of these snacks can be a hard-chew vegetable or fruit just to keep that good blood sugar going. Or the afternoon snack can also be a soft-chew fruit, such as a half grapefruit, a peach, a slice of ripe melon, berries, an orange, or a plum, because blood sugar is now controlled and you only have to maintain it. Once your blood sugar levels are balanced, you can have a greater range of choice in your diet, since you only have to *maintain* your good blood sugar—not create it. (See soft-chew choices on page 91.)

Here's an important note: You don't have to eat two afternoon snacks. If you plan on eating dinner at six P.M. and you ate lunch at one P.M. and your first afternoon snack at four P.M., then just call up and make reservations.

You can forget that second hard or soft chew. But make certain that you are actually eating your meal within three hours. If you're going to a restaurant that's notorious for long waits, have that second snack as you head downtown. It would be a shame to lose that good-blood-sugar feeling at the end of the day—and harmful foods become much too tempting.

If you're not eating until eight, it's *vital* that you have that second snack to keep your blood-sugar level balanced.

HARD-CHEW SAVVY

There's a fine line between eating extra vegetable hard chews and nibbling baby carrots the whole day through. Do eat them as you need them, but in the right amounts and within the right time. Nibbling carrots or string beans or cauliflower florettes all day might be a healthy, low-cal alternative to the vending machine, but it can dilute the effect of your goal: to raise and stabilize good blood sugar on the 5-Day Miracle Diet. Eat more vegetables certainly, in addition to your hard chew, if you need them. And, yes, nibble them at your desk. Just don't spread your scheduled hard-chew snacks out throughout the whole day. Have a specific amount at a specific time rather than unconsciously reaching for the plastic bag while you work.

ADELE PUHN'S STEP 6: TRY TO EAT DINNER NO LATER THAN EIGHT O'CLOCK AT NIGHT— BUT EARLIER IS BETTER.

As with lunch, dinner consists of vegetables and protein. All the veggies can be cooked and have a soft-chew texture.

It is not necessary to have a hard chew at night. (See food choices starting on page 81.) If you haven't had starch at lunch, you can have it now, with dinner. *Bread is a lunch-time option only* and may not be saved for other meals. However, bread may be included for dinner in place of the carbo choices listed. You decide. Men can have potatoes, beans, grains, or other starchy carbohydrates every day—unless the carbohydrates are a part of a vegetarian meal; then twice a day is fine. Women can have them every other day—unless they are a part of a vegetarian meal; then a daily starchy carbohydrate is fine.

Whether you are a man or a woman, a vegetarian meal must consist of starch and vegetables. But you don't have to be a vegetarian to enjoy a vegetarian meal. You can make dinner a vegetarian one—*if* you had protein at lunch. (See "Vegetarian Dining" on page 83.) Dinner should be your last meal of the day. And if you're in good blood sugar, you won't even miss dessert or that nighttime snack. But if eat you must, pick something from the "Quick Fix" list on page 92 until you feel stabilized. Just keep in mind that eating late at night is not a good idea; your body cannot digest food as quickly, and insufficient digestion results in greater fat storage.

In the first few weeks, while your blood sugar is getting balanced (or rebalanced, if you've been in a state of bad blood sugar for whatever reason), these "Quick Fixes" will help keep cravings at bay. Instead of sugar or alcohol, which keep cravings strong, you'll "hit" on a food that will satisfy the need for the moment without a rebound effect—even if you're eating more calories than usual. (And calories don't count on the 5-Day Miracle Diet, because if counting calories worked, the whole world would be thin!)

Sometimes dinner can be tricky. Suppose you're going out or it's a Saturday night and you're not planning on eating until nine or ten. (But do keep in mind that it's only in Barcelona that this is the rule. In our country it's the exception—and if you always eat dinner late, it's not going to help you lose weight or maintain good blood sugar.)

For those times when you do dine out late, make sure you have your timed afternoon snacks before dinner (as many as necessary to keep the "every three hours" rule). You will also have to "own" the idea that you are going to be needy the next day. Eating late at night weakens your blood-sugar-level balance, so you will need "intensive correction" (more hard-chew snacks) for the next day or two. It's times like these that "Quick Fixes" can come in handy.

THE PROOF IS IN THE EATING

As reported in the *New England Journal of Medicine,* a diet that included snacks was more effective in controlling cholesterol levels and insulin secretion than a standard three-meals-a-day diet.

I remember Sam and "The Banana That Came to the Meeting." Sam had already lost fifteen pounds on the 5-Day Miracle Diet. He'd been on the program for over a month and felt comfortable with it. But the night before an important meeting he had to take some out-of-town clients to dinner. Their plane got in late and Sam didn't have dinner until ten P.M. He'd brought carrots to the airport, so he had his timed snacks, but the late dinner still threw him slightly off balance. The next day he woke up groggier than usual. He got to the meeting and noticed, as if it was sitting in the chair next to him, a banana amid a platter of fruit on the conference table. It was calling to him, waving to him, blowing kisses at him. He went for the banana with a passion, never seeing the juicy apples and pears that were in the fruit bowl as well. When I asked him why he ate the banana, he merely shrugged. It was there. He had an overwhelming need to have it. The other fruit was invisible.

Unfortunately the banana kept his blood sugar off-kilter; it took a few days to get back on track. If Sam had grabbed a Quick Fix "hit," he'd have gotten back in balance much sooner—and he'd have regained his vitality and energy much faster.

PASSION-FOOD TRIGGERS: RAISINS AND OTHERS

These fruits can *never* be used as hard or soft chews. Nor can they be used as Quick Fixes. They are too sweet and hypoglycemic—and can play havoc with your blood-sugar levels. Think of them as Extras, for that twice-a-week "Foods You Adore" time. P.S. I promise that when you are in good blood sugar, you won't even realize these exist!

Bananas	Pineapple
Cherries	Honeydew
Grapes	Papaya
Dried fruits	Mango

If you spurn the passion-food triggers, you will be in good blood sugar. You'll be able to eat your dinner and call it a day—without missing a beat. Enjoy some exotic grains, such as couscous, and some unusual vegetables, such as baby eggplants or yellow peppers. Try a grilled tuna steak or tofu marinated in garlic. Experiment. You won't be bored and your body will thank you for its good health!

That's all there is to it! Your blood sugar is stabilized and you've maintained it throughout the evening. You're ready to sleep soundly and peacefully the whole night through.

In the beginning all this might sound like a foreign language because you are not accustomed to thinking about foods in this way. You will most likely walk around with this book in your attaché case, on your night table, in your desk drawer. But after five days you won't even need to look at the 5-Day Miracle Diet anymore. Why? Because you will be so certain of what you are supposed to do—thanks to the clear thinking that comes from being in good blood sugar and the experience of being on the program itself. You'll feel like a pro and ready to "own" the diet, to make it a part of who you are and what you are—for good.

EXTRA, EXTRA!

Once you are in consistent good blood sugar (which usually takes five days), the "fun" part begins: selective "Extras." I insist my clients eat something they adore once or twice a week—*as little as possible to make them happy*. You might find that some weeks you'll need to eat more of that Boston cream pie, while other weeks one bite will do. Whatever. As long as it does the job. It's all a part of owning the 5-Day Miracle Diet and incorporating it into your life.

TIMING IS EVERYTHING

Here are some timetables to help illustrate your options concerning when to eat your meals and your snacks—regardless of whether you are a night owl, an early bird, or a person who likes to sleep late on weekends.

EARLY RISER

7:30	Wake up	7:30	Wake up
8:00	Breakfast	8:00	Breakfast
10:00	Hard-chew snack	10:00	Hard-chew snack
12:00	Second hard-chew snack	12:00	Lunch
1:00	Lunch	3:00	Soft- or hard-chew snack
4:00	Soft- or hard-chew snack	6:00	Soft- or hard-chew snack
6:00	Dinner	7:00	Dinner

A SNOOZER

8:30	Wake up	8:30	Wake up
9:00	Breakfast	9:00	Breakfast
11:00	Hard-chew snack	11:00	Hard-chew snack
1:00	Lunch	1:00	Lunch
4:00	Soft- or hard-chew snack	4:00	Soft- or hard-chew snack
7:00	Soft- or hard-chew snack	7:00	Dinner
8:00	Dinner		

MORNING EXERCISER

6:30	Wake up	6:30	Wake up
6:45	Exercise	6:45	Exercise
7:30	Breakfast	7:30	Breakfast
9:30	Hard-chew snack	9:00	Hard-chew snack
11:30	Second hard-chew snack	11:00	Second hard-chew snack

12:30	Lunch	1:00	Lunch
3:30	Soft- or hard-chew snack	4:00	Soft- or hard-chew snack
6:00	Dinner	7:00	Dinner

MOON WATCHER

10:00	Wake up	10:00	Wake up
10:30	Breakfast	10:30	Breakfast
12:30	Hard-chew snack	12:30	Hard-chew snack
2:30	Lunch	2:30	Lunch
5:30	Soft- or hard-chew snack	5:30	Soft- or hard-chew snack
8:30	Dinner	7:00	Soft- or hard-chew snack
		9:30	Dinner

WEEKEND SLEEPER

We all need to live on a circadian rhythm. If you are an "early riser" five days a week and enjoy sleeping in on the weekend, you can throw your body all out of balance if you suddenly "shock" it with a different eating rhythm. The solution? Lunch by 12:30—no matter what. Have your hard chews within two hours of lunch. Remember, there's no such thing as brunch!

10:00	Wake up	8:00	Wake up
10:30	Breakfast	8:30	Breakfast
12:30	Lunch	10:30	Hard-chew snack
2:30	Hard-chew snack	11:30	Lunch *(not brunch)*
4:30	Soft- or hard-chew snack	2:30	Soft- or hard-chew snack
6:30	Soft- or hard-chew snack (or dinner)	5:00	Soft- or hard-chew snack
8:00	Dinner	7:00	Soft- or hard-chew snack
		8:00	Dinner

IT'S SUNDAY AND YOU ARE TO MEET SOME FRIENDS
FOR BRUNCH AT 11:30 . . .

10:30	Wake up
11:00	Hard-chew snack
11:30	Breakfast (which everyone else is calling brunch)
1:30–2:00	Lunch
Every two hours	Soft- or hard-chew snack
By 7:00	Dinner

As you can see, there is no such thing as cheating on
the 5-Day Miracle Diet. You can have whatever "Extras"
you decide. Some weeks it might be only the one or two
"Extras." Other weeks there might be, say, several birth-
days, or a holiday, or a cruise. In this case you might
even have "Extras" for seven days. (This is of course the
exception, not the rule!) But that's not cheating. You
know what you are doing; you are making a conscious
decision to eat something you adore and enjoy it to the
hilt. The only cheating on the 5-Day Miracle Diet occurs
when you aren't dealing with your food, when you let the
food control you, when you don't own the diet and incor-
porate it into your life.

Your "Extra" can be a hot fudge sundae, a burger
platter, a Caesar salad, a fabulous pasta dish, a spicy
Bloody Mary—anything that makes you feel good and
not deprived. But remember, "as little as possible to feel
happy." Do *not* eat a "trigger" food, such as frozen yogurt
for lunch, or, say, a bag of chips for an afternoon snack.
These are called "Extras." These foods should be eaten
only once or twice a week—and *always* in addition to
your regular, timed diet plan. If you remove your control
snacks and hit on an "Extra" that will drop your blood
sugar, you'll be playing a game of Double Jeopardy.
Without the right foods behind it, your body will lose its

foundation. You'll be in the bad-blood-sugar basement without a light—or a banister to help you up the stairs.

IF YOU CAN'T BEAT THEM, JOIN THEM

Absolute abstinence is easier for overweight people than reasonable eating—but only in the short run. Eventually the "white-knuckled" approach will have you grabbing for that cookie jar. Desserts, luscious meals, crunchy snacks are here to stay—and the best way to face them is with relish—in good blood sugar and as a planned Extra!

ADELE PUHN'S FOUR RULES OF SELECTIVITY

You must follow my Four Rules of Selectivity when you decide on an "Extra" in order to ensure weight loss and balanced blood-sugar levels.

1. *You must be in good blood sugar.* If not, the rest of the rules won't work. The low-blood-sugar ventriloquist will be speaking for you!
2. *The food you choose must be appropriate.* It must make you happy, and eating it should be an exciting event. For example, a delicious dessert in a fabulous restaurant while dining with good friends is an excellent choice. Scarfing down a box of Girl Scout cookies while standing at the kitchen counter is not.
3. *The food must be something you really, really love.* It is not good enough to eat something just because you like it and it is available. We like too much and there's *too much* available. And frankly when you're in bad blood sugar, everything is "adorable."

4. *You should eat just enough to make you happy—
whatever that amount may be.* Remember, there's no
cheating. You can have the same food in a few days.
However, remember, too, that if you eat a large portion of a particularly sugary, carbo-laden "Extra," you
will be held accountable for it the next day. But that
is okay. You "own" the diet. Recognize the signs of
"blood-sugar vulnerability" and stay with your program. You'll be fine within forty-eight hours—and
the "Extra" was worth it!

On the other hand, you can be like Sondra, one of my
clients who "lived" for her "Extras." From week to week
she thought about what she was going to eat as an "Extra." It got to the point where she would eat the most boring, tasteless meals and snacks—just so that she could
load up on ice cream on Sunday. She wouldn't eat grilled
salmon steak because it was too fatty. She wouldn't eat
roasted vegetables because they were cooked with a
pinch of oil. She stayed away from unsweetened peanut
butter and avoided pasta, rice, even whole wheat rolls.
Instead she religiously stuck to rice cakes, tofu, steamed
vegetables, and plain broiled fish and chicken.

Her diet became so boring, so deprived that, sure
enough, one week, her "Extra," a Caesar salad, turned
into a roast beef dinner with all the trimmings, pie à
la mode for dessert, and, once she got to her apartment,
an entire box of doughnuts she'd purchased on the
way home.

I'm happy to report that Sondra realized that her an-
ticipation was playing havoc with the food sensualist
within her—ultimately overpowering her blood-sugar
balance. She was no more in control than when she was
continuously in bad blood sugar. She's stopped living for
her "Extras" and lives for today. She now enjoys every

meal she has, *including* her "Extras." She's in good blood sugar and losing weight.

How can there be these "Extras" on a diet program? Simple. Because you, like my clients, will be in good blood sugar, your uncontrollable cravings will be absent. You won't overeat—and you will enjoy every bite of your food. You won't gain weight!

"That's it?" you say, incredulously. Well, yes and no. That's the basic diet. But there are three nonfood elements that will ensure your success.

THE THREE BASIC PUHN PRINCIPLES TO ENSURE 5-DAY MIRACLE DIET PLAN SUCCESS

1. Eat at specific times during the day.
2. Eat specific types of food.
3. Eat specific combinations and textures of food.

THE FOOD DIARY

If there's one single thing besides blood-sugar control you can do on your program to guarantee long-term success, it's the food diary. I know, you've heard it before. Well, you haven't heard it from me. Write down what you eat. And I have to tell you that all of my successful clients have kept a food diary.

First of all, this diet is unique, and timing is very important. Since you are not familiar with it, especially in the beginning, it's crucial to write down the *times* you eat your meals and your snacks—and *what* you eat.

This way you can analyze your successes—and your relapses. By writing down the foods you eat, the times, and the way you feel, you can identify the situations that have the potential for temptation and work out resolutions. Here's an example:

Don, a busy advertising executive, was stuck in a meeting way past the time for his second snack of the morning. More than four hours passed before he was able to have lunch. The meeting threw his timing out of whack—and his blood sugar. He was no longer losing weight and he had all the symptoms of bad blood sugar: crankiness, a lack of energy, cravings, and an inability to concentrate. By looking at his food diary, he was able to identify the problem: meetings that run late at least twice a week. And he was able to solve the problem: Eat a hard chew *before* the meeting—even if it is too early—just to cover the possibility he may have to stay in the meeting past his usual twelve-thirty lunchtime. This timing will keep him protected and he will maintain his good blood sugar.

The food diary is not a report card. It's a workbook designed specifically for you. Think of it as a commitment to the program: "Perfect" or not, you will write down everything you eat. Indeed, if you don't write down what you've eaten, you can forget, or what I call "go blank." It makes for great bad-blood-sugar excuses—and *fathead* self-sabotage that makes you completely "blameless" and unaccountable for the food you eat.

I had a client who traveled a great deal. He couldn't be bothered with a food diary; he always told me what he ate, week after week. He knew the times to eat, he always grabbed a hard chew, and he never ate after dinner. However, he wasn't losing weight. I told him to think really hard about what he'd eaten—just yesterday.

"Nothing I shouldn't have," he replied.

I waited.

"Hmm . . ." He began to think.

Suddenly he remembered: There were the nuts on the plane. How could he have forgotten? And then there was the banana in the hotel room fridge. And the chocolate bar he grabbed at the airport while he waited for a taxi . . .

No wonder he couldn't lose weight! He unconsciously "blanked" out the food he ate by not writing things down in his diary.

The food diary is a great tool. You didn't lose weight one week? Look at your food diary. Perhaps it's because you ate four adored "Extras" instead of two. You feel a craving coming on? Look at your food diary. Perhaps it's because you've been teasing yourself with only one snack in the morning and none in the afternoon. You had a great week and you feel marvelous? Look at your food diary. You stayed in good blood sugar. It's right there in black and white. And if you did it once, you can do it again!

There's another component to the food diary. (See the blank food-diary sample in appendix B.) It's the section called "Comments." This is the place for you to write your thoughts—whatever they may be on that particular day. The food diary is for you and only you. It's there to help you lose weight. Yes, you can see the biochemical aspects right away if you write in your food diary. But if you use the "Comments" section, you can also see the psychological underpinnings that can come into play.

🢒 🢒 🢒 🢒 🢒 🢒 🢒 🢒 🢒 🢒

"OFF THE TRACK" FOOD DIARY SAMPLE

WEDNESDAY, 12/18
   8:00 A.M.: Breakfast: cottage cheese and pita
               bread
  10:00 A.M.: 4 cookies
  11:00 A.M.: 1 apple
   1:00 P.M.: Lunch: pita bread and turkey
   6:00 P.M.: 1 apple
   8:00 P.M.: Dinner: hot and sour soup, twice-
               cooked pork, fried rice

Comment on the Day: It was really hard. I feel
discouraged. Makes me want to eat more.

Adele's Comment: I could see it coming. The next
day this client had her breakfast, Post bran flakes,
and then . . . blank. She'd eaten cookies instead
of her hard-chew snack. It made sense. She had
lunch before getting in her two hard chews—an
apple at ten, perhaps, and a handful of string
beans at twelve. She also missed her veggies at
lunch—a vital component to the noontime meal
because they provide a slow release of glucose
during digestion and help maintain good blood
sugar. Plus she missed her hard chew at lunch,
which would have tied the ribbon on her good
blood sugar. By the time dinner rolled around,
her body chemistry had gone up and down. She
was helpless. I'm pleased that she didn't eat *more*
Chinese food at dinner!
    There were many reasons for this "technical
interference": forgetting her snacks, eating late
at night, too big portions, and eating restricted
food.
    The next day was encouraging: She started her
day with a slice of whole-grain bread and a slice
of nonfat cheese. She ate a hard-chew snack
within two hours of breakfast. She was on the

right track. Even better, she went over her food diary at her next visit and discussed some of the psychological *fathead* issues facing her: stress at work and a child in trouble at school, problems that made her turn to food for self-destruction, as "a weapon of choice."

"ON TRACK" FOOD DIARY SAMPLE

8:00 A.M.:	Breakfast: cottage cheese and eight-grain bread
10:00 A.M.:	Apple
12:00 P.M.:	2 carrots
12:30 P.M.:	Lunch: 3 ounces tuna (packed in water), 1 slice whole-wheat bread, raw broccoli
3:30 P.M.:	2 tangerines
6:30 P.M.:	Broccoli and cauliflower
7:30 P.M.:	Dinner: turkey burger, spinach, broccoli rabe, salad with olive oil and balsamic vinegar

Comment on the day: Great! The tangerines were delicious. I'm very energetic.

Adele's Comments: This client has lost a total of forty-five pounds. He continues to follow my food plan, and his food cravings have all but disappeared. There is no "technical interference" between his body's chemistry and his blood-sugar level. He continues to work on the psychological *fathead* issues to help maintain his weight loss.

My clients come to see me on a weekly basis in the beginning of the program. The first thing we do, after a quick weighing in, is look at the food diary they've kept. We begin to talk. Remember, cravings are 75 percent physiological—and 25 percent psychological. It is important for you to understand the ramifications of the *fathead*, these internal and external saboteurs that come into play when low blood sugar is no longer speaking for you.

Since you're not coming in and speaking to me, the "Comments" give you a chance to write down your feelings and analyze them in the privacy of your home. "My boyfriend's parents came to visit and I was nervous . . . and I ate." "I had a big presentation at work. I was up all night. The cravings were talking to me." Or simply: "I feel empowered! I never felt so free!"

The *fathead* is so important that I've devoted an entire chapter to it later on. But for now suffice it to say that your food diary should never be farther away from you than your fork or spoon.

SHOOTING THE SCALE

Forget that can't-wait, ohmigod, let's-get-this-over-with, will-it-help-if-I-take-off-my-earrings/watch/necklace/belt process called Weighing In.

Shooting the scale. Period. It's done fast and furiously. And it's over within a minute. Shooting the scale minimizes your focus on numbers. Stop thinking in "pounds" so that you aren't driven to weigh yourself every day—and you aren't deciding to binge because on one particular day you just so happened not to lose weight. You don't want the scale to tell you how to feel or what to eat.

Frankly I don't care what you weigh. I know that the scale is a good benchmark to see the progress we're making, but it can also be a trap. I remember an old *Twilight Zone* episode years back. A man had gone to Las Vegas and had become enamored of the slot machines. He eventually became so obsessed that not only did he lose all his money but the slot machine came to life and slammed its way, all shiny and jangly, into his hotel room.

Your scale can become that slot machine, an obsession that follows you everywhere. It can take over your life. True, your scale is a way of gauging weight loss, but so is an easier-fitting pair of pants. My feeling? What you weigh is less important than how you feel and how you look.

Besides, there are so many variables at work on your weight. Your menstrual cycle. The muscle mass that develops after you begin working out—which weighs more than fat. Sodium and water retention from a particularly salty meal. And, believe it or not, getting into good blood sugar, possibly for the first time in your life, is much more of a "high" than those two or four pounds per week—although you will have that, too!

SCALING DOWN

Forget the scale except for once a week, when you weigh yourself in the same clothes in the same place at the same time. And instead of concentrating on those numbers, spend your week noticing that your clothes are feeling looser.

Other hints: If you look in the mirror with all your clothes off, you're looking for trouble. You'll zero in on your imperfections. No one likes the way he or she looks! Instead, glance at your reflection as you pass a store window, dressed for work. Or turn around in front of your mirror wearing that favorite blouse or jeans you hadn't been able to wear for years. Look at the confidence. The slim contours you show the world. The health and energy that positively exude from you. How poised, strong, and confident you look! *That's* what is important—not the numbers on the scale.

FOOD FACT OF LIFE: WHAT YOU ATE ON SUNDAY MIGHT NOT SHOW UP UNTIL TUESDAY . . .

EVEN IF YOU STAYED IN GOOD BLOOD SUGAR ALL DAY MONDAY!

It happens to all of us: We get sidetracked. We choose to eat or drink something laden with carbs or sugar. We celebrate. We "miss a beat." Just remember:

- What you eat in the morning will affect you in the evening.
- What you eat on Monday will affect you on Tuesday—and possibly Wednesday.
- When you are in good blood sugar and you "miss a beat," the effects will become very clear—and you'll get back into the rhythm with more hard chews, extra activity, and the knowledge that in a short time you'll be dancing with the best of them!
- Sometimes seeing a weight gain after a day or two of 5-Day Miracle Diet eating is discouraging. It's hard to believe that the champagne and caviar you had on Sunday took so long to catch up with your body. The occasional result? Dropping out. All the more reason to "shoot the scale" only once a week—and not put too much importance on those numbers. They are only powerful if you let them be!

EXERCISE

No, I didn't forget the stretching, the exhilarating aerobics, the dancing, walking, biking, just-getting-off-the-couch-and-moving part of any diet plan. I know people in bad blood sugar have enough trouble just getting through the day. I prefer introducing exercise in the 5-Day Miracle Diet after my clients have stabilized their blood-sugar level.

But once you are in good blood sugar, exercise becomes an important element in your weight-loss success. (And since you now have so much vitality and energy, you're actually going to *want* to move!)

In fact I've designed my own personal "fifteen-minute stretch" to get your good blood sugar going in the morning—as well as suggestions to fit exercise into your life. I'll be going over all of this in chapter 8, but for now simply think about it. Think about taking the stairs instead of the elevator. Think about parking a little farther away from the store. Think about getting off the bus five or six blocks after your actual stop. Think about walking instead of taking the car.

Yes, just think about it. You're starting a new way of being, a new way of life, that will make you feel terrific. Your body will change—and so will your attitude. But for now go slow. It will happen.

PUHN-ATTUNED HEALTH MUSTS

For maximum health benefits and weight loss, here are a few more "Puhn-Attuned Health Musts" incorporated into the 5-Day Miracle Diet.

*Healthy Rule 1: Try to Drink at Least Eight Glasses of
Water a Day*

Fresh from the tap, if safe. Distilled. Sparkling. Lemon-
or lime-flavored. Seltzered. Water, any way you take it,
is imperative. Not only does water carry toxic waste out
of your body, it also nourishes your cells and keeps your
body's organs running smoothly. Most diets suggest between six to eight 8-ounce glasses a day, but the latest research shows that between eight and twelve glasses a day
are best. This does not include herb teas or decaffeinated
drinks. It's water—the most efficient vehicle for elimination ever created.

▲   ▲   ▲   ▲   ▲   ▲   ▲   ▲   ▲

WATER, WATER EVERYWHERE

Water is good for you. Period. But the old school
of diet thought spoke of water easing appetite.
Nonsense. Water flushes out your system; it
keeps you hydrated. But it does not fill you up.
Staying in good blood sugar will curb those appetite cravings—not water.

However, if you are one of those people who
produce too much digestive acids, this overproduction can mimic hunger. When you drink a
lot of water, these digestive acids that mimic
hunger get diluted—which gives you the illusion
of satiation. But in reality you're really just dilut-
ing these acids.

▼   ▼   ▼   ▼   ▼   ▼   ▼   ▼   ▼

Some ways to get in your water?

- Try a cup of hot water with fresh lemon when you first
  get up in the morning. It helps digestion and elimination, and it refreshes you.
- Drink a glass of water before each meal.

- Keep a large bottle of water in your office. It's easier to drink at room temperature. You can sip from it all day long without even thinking about it. Or, just as easily, chug it down in one fell swoop and be done with it.
- Drink a glass of water as soon as you wake up.
- Drink a full glass of water along with your vitamin supplements.

COFFEE TO GO

We all know that herbal teas are healthier for our systems, but if you need your coffee, go ahead and drink it with a little skim or 1% milk—as long as you don't use sugar or artificial sweeteners. Once you are in good blood sugar, I promise you won't be that committed to your coffee—which is why I'm not particularly concerned when people tell me they "can't live without their coffee" when they initially come in to see me. In the first few weeks just keep it down to a minimum, or try decaf in the afternoon.

Healthy Rule 2: Take a Multi-Vitamin-and-Mineral Supplement at Breakfast

Although my program consists of healthy foods that are high in vitamins and minerals and in amounts that are sound for your weight, there are still reasons why you should take supplements. Important reasons.

First of all, there's our lifestyle. Contrary to what we preach, our lives are not filled with "quality time." We work, we commute, we spend time with our family, we do our errands and chores, and, if we're lucky, we get a decent night's sleep. Many of us are like Paul, a financial whiz who keeps a packed suitcase of essential clothes and duplicate grooming items for last-minute business trips.

Our ancestors certainly didn't have late meetings, impossible deadlines, and commuter traffic. Unfortunately today's hectic, toxic environment makes for irregular eating patterns and additional stress—which places greater nutritional needs on our bodies. Only a vitamin-mineral supplement can fill in the gaps.

Then there's the way our food is grown. It's very different from the way it was grown on those idyllic local farms of yore. Much of what we eat is imported—and we have no control over its production or growth. It's an unfortunate fact: We live in a toxic world. The soil doesn't contain the nutrients it did long ago; the use of chemical fertilizers is widespread; the food that is produced can lack essential vitamins and minerals. For example, selenium, an important antioxidant that has been found in some studies to help prevent cancer, used to be abundant in our soil—which in turn made our foods, particularly garlic and onion, selenium-rich. No more. Today, without a multi-vitamin-and-mineral, you most likely won't get enough selenium. A case in point: In the Northeast, where the soil's selenium depletion is a known fact, cancer rates are quite high.

Add the fact that we are less physical and that our eating habits, as a nation, are more "fast food" than not, and you can see why a vitamin-mineral supplement is something you should take—even if you are on my healthy, balanced program.

PILL TALK

Your multi-vitamin-mineral should contain the following:

VITAMINS	PERCENTAGE OF RDA
Vitamin A (as beta-carotene), 10,000 IU	200%
Vitamin D, 400 IU	100%
Vitamin E, 60 IU	200%
Vitamin K, 60 mcg	*
Vitamin C, 120 mg	200%
Folic acid, 400 mcg	100%
Vitamin B1, 1.5 mg	100%
Vitamin B2, 2 mg	100%
Vitamin B6, 2 mg	100%
Vitamin B12, 6 mcg	100%
Pantothenic acid, 10 mg	100%
Biotin, 30 mcg	10%

MINERALS	PERCENTAGE OF RDA
Calcium, 162 mg	16%
Phosphorus, 109 mg	11%
Iodine, 150 mcg	100%
Iron, 9 mg	50%
Magnesium, 100 mg	25%
Copper, 3 mg	150%
Zinc, 22.5 mg	150%
Manganese, 2.5 mg	*
Potassium, 40 mg	*
Chromium, 100 mcg	*
Molybdenum, 25 mcg	*
Selenium, 45 mcg	*
Nickel, 5 mcg	*
Tin, 10 mcg	*
Silicon, 2 mcg	*
Vanadium, 10 mcg	*
Boron, 150 mcg	*

*RDA not established

Healthy Rule 3: Take a Calcium Pill Daily, Preferably at Bedtime

As you begin my program, you'll notice that there's no yogurt—and few milk products. There's a good reason for this. Yogurt, for example, is very glycemic. It's a predigestive protein, which makes it too easily absorbed, just like bagels, bananas, and white bread. It's healthy, but not to control your cravings or help you lose weight. And milk itself contains lactose—which can have the same properties as these highly glycemic foods. As I mentioned earlier, certain dairy products, especially "diet delights" such as frozen yogurt or ice milk, can trigger a chemical imbalance and deliver a craving to your system—while other milk products will provide extra fat.

Karla thought she was being virtuous when she ordered a plain frozen yogurt at lunch. After all, she figured, it was low in calories and it was good for her, too. And it tasted great!

However, no more than two hours after her yogurt lunch her body's ventriloquist began to speak to her: "Feed me. Feed me now." She ran down to the office cafeteria and bought a sandwich to eat at her desk. By the time dinner rolled around, she'd been completely taken over by her cravings. She ate pasta, Italian bread, and Gorgonzola cheese—which set back her bad blood sugar even more.

Frozen yogurt, as we now know, is a poor choice. There are other calcium-rich foods that contain less sugar and less of those "triggering," too-easily-digested enzymes that yogurt is laden with—and they do not come only in white liquid packages. Make sure you eat some of the foods listed in "Foods Rich in Calcium" to ensure you are meeting your calcium requirements every day.

FOODS RICH IN CALCIUM

Sardines (with bones)	3 oz.	372 mg of calcium
Skim milk	8 oz.	302 mg
Oysters	1 cup	226 mg
Farina	1 cup	189 mg
Canned salmon	3 oz.	150 mg
Spinach, cooked	1 cup	244 mg
Broccoli, cooked	1 cup	178 mg
Cottage cheese	½ cup	63 mg
Orange	1 med.	60 mg
Tofu	4 oz.	154 mg
Kale	1 cup	206 mg
Collards	1 cup	357 mg
Turnip greens	1 cup	267 mg
Bok choy	1 cup	116 mg
Soy milk	1 cup	146 mg

Be aware that calcium is a necessary nutrient and that we need different amounts at different stages of our lives. As a general rule I tell my clients to take one or two 200 mg calcium supplements. There are many varieties out there, but I prefer calcium citrate with magnesium. It doesn't have the same potential for toxicity as oyster-shell calcium, and the magnesium helps keep proper mineral balance. However, the combination of magnesium and calcium can disagree with some people. The magnesium is a stool softener and the calcium is a binder. I strongly recommend checking with your professional health practitioner to determine the correct type and dosage of calcium that's right for you.

DAILY CALCIUM REQUIREMENTS

Adolescents (16–19):	1,500 mg
Adults (men and women):	1,500 mg
Menopausal women:	1,800 mg
Pregnant/lactating women:	2,000 mg
Postmenopausal women:	1,800 mg

These amounts can be reached through a combination of calcium-rich foods and calcium supplements.

I also ask my clients to take their supplement at night. Calcium is a natural tranquilizer that stimulates the chemicals in your brain to relay the message: sleep. Your grandmother knew that warm cup of milk at night was as good as a lullaby!

MILK IS NOT ALWAYS YOUR BEST FRIEND

The commercials and the onslaught of articles that milk can help prevent osteoporosis can make anyone start gulping the stuff. But think again. It's calcium that does the trick, *not* the milk. In fact the recommended dose of calcium per day for women between age twenty-four and menopause is 1,500 milligrams. For postmenopausal women this number goes up to 1,800 milligrams. Milk, whether it be skim or whole, contains only 300 milligrams per 8-ounce glass. You have to drink a lot of milk to get the results—and you might find yourself with the side effects of lactose intolerance: a bloated feeling, gas, or heartburn.

Another good choice for calcium comes from your fresh produce—not your dairy section.

Supplements can supply you with the extra

milligrams you need per day. I suggest calcium citrate. Oyster-shell calcium can be contaminated by toxins in the sea.

❦ ❦ ❦ ❦ ❦ ❦ ❦ ❦ ❦

Healthy Rule 4: It's Okay to Use Fat—Sparingly

I actually encourage eating some unsaturated fats on my diet—up to three teaspoons a day. Remember, this is a reasonable diet and we all try to live in a reasonable world. Our body cannot manufacture all its essential fatty acids— and we *need* a certain amount of unsaturated fats in our diets for good health, shiny hair, glowing skin, and strong nails. A drop of canola oil or virgin olive oil on a salad can make all the difference between feeling you're eating a wonderful dish and feeling deprived. Brushing a cold-pressed oil on your vegetables before grilling them gives them a lush, full taste.

▲ ▲ ▲ ▲ ▲ ▲ ▲ ▲ ▲

PRESS ON

If you've ever seen the words *cold-pressed* or *virgin* on your olive oil bottle, it is not just an excuse to add expense. Cold-pressing is a process of manufacturing olive oil that actually makes it healthier.

All vegetables must be heated to release, or "press out," the oil that is later found on your grocery shelf. Unfortunately in order to release all the oil, they must be heated to extreme temperatures—which not only reduces any nutritional value but also creates the dangerous "free radicals" we've heard so much about. These free radicals have a molecular structure that contains an extra electron, which has magnetic capabilities that make it highly clingable and malleable. So strongly reactive are these free radicals that they have been implicated in the development of certain cancers, heart disease, stroke, and aging. But cold-pressed olive oil uses much lower temperatures to extract its oils, and nutrients are thus saved and free radicals kept at bay.

I don't suggest measuring your fat; simply use your judgment. A small spoonful at lunch. A dollop on your fork, brushed on your salad. It's there, it's good for you—and it's not as if you're eating deep-fried chicken, which is loaded with cholesterol and saturated fat.

FAT FACT

Did you know that eating fat actually stimulates the burning of stored fat in your body? It also satiates your appetite. But it's a fine balance. Too much fat and it hangs around too long in your gut. The result? Low, low, bad blood sugar.

You need to address the food sensualist in you; you have to tailor your diet to appeal to your senses. Otherwise, sooner or later, your psychological needs will overcome your physiological stability and you'll be back in bad-blood-sugar land again.

PIZZA, PIZZA

Yes, you can have pizza on the 5-Day Miracle Diet. Once a week, feel free to indulge. The hard cheese on one slice "saves" your blood-sugar balance. The crust counts as a starch, so the starch rules apply: Have one slice for either lunch or dinner. And *always* have a salad with your pizza. Remember, veggies are supposed to make up the bulk of your meal to help stabilize your blood sugar.

If you want more than one slice, consider it done . . . as an "Extra."

❧   ❧   ❧   ❧   ❧   ❧   ❧   ❧   ❧

Healthy Rule 5: Limit Salt

Okay, okay. You've heard this one before. We use too much salt. The American Heart Association recommends less than 3,000 mg of salt per day for a healthy diet—and less if you have high blood pressure or any other heart condition.

I have found that once they've begun my diet, people actually want less salt. Their taste buds come awake and they find baby carrots sweet, an apple an incredible treat, the use of fresh herbs and spices exhilarating. I do not encourage the use of salt because of its relationship to high blood pressure. Although not definitely proven, salt has been found to stimulate high blood pressure and in turn heart disease. *Always* follow your physician's instructions regarding salt, especially if you have hypertension.

For those clients who do not have blood pressure problems and who can't imagine life without salt, I don't make a big issue about it—especially in the first few weeks. But I do suggest the following:

- Tasting your food before adding salt.
- Using little or no salt for cooking.
- Experimenting with a shake of herbs and spices instead of a shake of salt. Two good ones to try: fines herbes, which has a subtle, sweet taste, and herbes de Provence, a hearty spice that is wonderful with tomato sauces and soups.

A CONVERSATION ABOUT CHOLESTEROL

Cholesterol is not necessarily a dirty word. A waxy substance that is manufactured by our bodies, it is vital for many of our systems to function. But there is the problem of too much of a good thing. Too much food of animal origin, and cholesterol can build up in our arteries and clog them up.

Basically cholesterol is carried throughout our bloodstream by lipoproteins, particles of protein and fat that are produced in the liver. The lipoprotein that delivers the cholesterol to the various organs is called LDL—low-density lipoprotein. This is also called "bad" cholesterol because, if it builds up and is not removed or processed by our cells, the cholesterol and fat in the LDL comes to rest on artery walls, clogging them and causing heart attacks and stroke.

HDL, or high-density lipoprotein, is the "good" cholesterol. This lipoprotein carries the excess cholesterol and its waste back to the liver for more processing or for elimination. It acts like a vacuum cleaner, picking up the remnants left on the artery walls by the LDL, keeping our arteries open and clean and healthy.

A buildup of LDL can come from your genes. It can also come from eating too much cholesterol-rich foods, such as meats and liver, or from saturated fats.

Unsaturated fats, however, can actually promote the production of HDL, or at least keep LDL build-up to a minimum. Polyunsaturated fats can lower *total* cholesterol levels, both the bad LDL and the good HDL. Monounsaturated fats, such as canola oil and olive oil, lower only LDL cholesterol, leaving the good HDL cholesterol intact.

One more note: Exercise, from walking to swimming, has been found to increase levels of HDL.

IN A NUTSHELL: THE 5-DAY MIRACLE DIET PLAN

1. Eat breakfast within a half hour of waking up (forty-five minutes if you exercise in the morning).
2. Breakfast consists of a protein and a bread or, on alternate days, cereal and enough skim or 1% milk to cover.
3. Eat your first hard-chew snack within two hours of beginning breakfast.
4. Eat your second hard-chew snack within the next two hours if it isn't yet time for lunch.
5. Try to eat lunch by one P.M. (especially early risers). Lunch should consist of protein and vegetables (plus one hard-chew vegetable to tie the bow on your good blood sugar), or a vegetarian meal. Salad with a bit of oil is always a good choice. Bread is optional.
6. Afternoon snacks are three hours apart. They can be eaten sooner but not farther apart. You can eat soft-chew fruits at this time. Either one or two snacks will fit in before dinner.
7. Dinner always includes vegetables and proteins, or a vegetarian meal. Add whole grains, starchy vegetables, potatoes, or beans in the following way: Men can eat these starches every day, women only on alternate days—either for lunch *or* dinner, not both (unless you are eating a vegetarian meal).
8. Lunch and dinner should be composed of 30 to 40 percent vegetables. This includes salad.
9. Do not have pasta more than twice a week, and only at dinner.
10. Try to have one vegetarian meal a day. It's good for your health.
11. Take a multi-vitamin-mineral pill in the morning.
12. Take a calcium supplement before you go to sleep.

13. Don't forget your "Extras." After you are in good blood sugar, enjoy one or two foods a week that you absolutely adore.
14. Keep a food diary.

That's it! You now have the tools to begin your own 5-Day Miracle Diet. There's nothing left to do but to "walk inside my office, take a seat, and begin . . ."

THE 5-DAY MIRACLE DIET FOODS

THE GOOD BLOOD SUGAR (GBS) PROTEIN CHOICES

Meats should be baked, grilled, broiled, microwaved, poached, or steamed. You can use a small amount of unsaturated fat for stir-frying and light sautéing. Remove the skin of all chicken before eating; it holds the most calories and fat. (In a typical whole chicken that weighs three pounds, the meat has about 800 calories—and the skin an astonishing 1,900 calories!) Do not add bread crumbs or coatings before cooking. Experiment with vinegar-based marinades and different spices. The proteins with the least amounts of unhealthy fat are tofu, tempeh, and fish. Proteins that are high in saturated fat and cholesterol should be eaten in limited quantities. They are noted with an asterisk. *People who have high cholesterol, hypertension, or have been told by their medical professional to cut down on their cholesterol for any other reason should especially stay away from those foods with an asterisk.*

FISH

Bass	Octopus
Bay scallops	Pike
Bluefish	Pompano
Catfish	Rainbow trout
Cod	Salmon, canned and
Eel	drained, or fresh
Flounder	Sardines, packed in
Grouper	water or tomato
Haddock	sauce, drained
Halibut	Swordfish
Herring	Tilefish
Mackerel	Tuna, fresh or canned
Monkfish	in spring water

SHELLFISH

Clams	Lobster
Crabmeat	Mussels
Crayfish	Oysters

MEATS AND POULTRY

- Beef, ground, round, sirloin, roast beef, flank: USDA Select or Choice
- Chicken (white meat), without skin
- Chicken (dark meat), without skin
- Cornish hens, without skin
- Deli chicken slice
- Deli turkey slice
- Duck, without skin
- Ham, lean
- Lamb, chops or roast (1 small chop is a portion)
- Pork, chops, lean medallions, roast
- Turkey (white meat), without skin
- Turkey (dark meat), without skin
- Veal, ground or chops

CHEESES

All cheeses should be *low-fat* versions, with no more than 60 percent fat per 1-ounce serving. All cheese is higher in fat than other proteins. Limit to twice a week. If you must limit your salt intake, be wary of cheese.

- Alpine Lace (low-fat brand name)
- American
- Cheddar
- Colby
- Edam
- Farmer (low-fat in regular package)
- Feta (low-fat in regular package)
- Fontina
- Gouda
- Gruyère
- Havarti
- Jarlsberg
- Monterey Jack
- Mozzarella, part-skim
- Muenster
- Parmesan
- Provolone
- Ricotta, skim-milk
- Swiss

MISCELLANEOUS

Because unsweetened peanut butter is a high-fat food, limit it to twice a week—*counted with any hard cheese you might eat.* (In other words, your total intake of peanut butter and hard cheese combined cannot be more than twice a week, either one serving peanut butter and one serving cheese, or two servings peanut butter, or two servings hard cheese.) Avoid reduced-fat peanut butter; it contains sugar.

⅓–½ cup no-fat cottage cheese or whey cheese
Egg substitutes
3 egg whites
1 or 2 eggs

*2–6 teaspoons peanut butter, unsweetened (limited)
1–4 ounces tempeh

VEGETARIAN DINING

Choose vegetarian meals as often as you desire.
I recommend eating at least one vegetarian
meal a day. This can include:

- A medium baked potato with salad and/or
  other vegetables
- Bean or vegetable soup (with chunks of
  potato in the soup) and salad
- Pasta (half an order or a small full order) and
  vegetables with a salad (twice a week and at
  dinner only)
- 1 cup (women) to 1½ cups (men) brown
  rice, millet, quinoa, or couscous served with
  steamed vegetables and/or salad

Or experiment. Use the following vegetarian proteins combined with at least 1 cup of grain:

- ½ cup lentils for women, ⅔–¾ cup for men
- 1 cup soy milk
- 2 ounces soy cheese
- 3 ounces tofu
- ½ cup beans, such as garbanzo, pinto, black,
  kidney, soy, and white beans for women;
  ⅔–¾ cup for men.

If you are a vegetarian, simply adjust your proteins to include beans and starchy vegetable at
both lunch and dinner. Always have your proteins with a grain and a variety of vegetables. Try
to have tofu, soy cheeses, and other soy products, as they are high in protein.

FRUIT CHOICES

Fruit has many vitamins and nutrients necessary for good health. Plus fruit tastes good—and it supplies a healthy "sugar" hit if you feel a craving coming on. Fruits can be used as soft-chew snacks, eaten at scheduled times and in correct amounts during the afternoon. Fruits other than apples and pears can also be eaten as an extra snack if you weigh over 200 pounds. But try not to eat your fruits after dinner; it can play havoc with your blood sugar.

Fruit should be eaten raw or, if frozen, unsweetened and without any syrup or juice. Serving size is one medium fruit, except where indicated.

Apple	½ grapefruit
4 small apricots	Nectarine
⅔ cup blueberries, raspberries, or blackberries	Orange
	Peach
	Pear
½ small cantaloupe	2 small plums
Chinese apple	1¼ cups strawberries
2 small tangerines	1 kiwi

STARCH/CARBOHYDRATE CHOICES

Cereals, grains, breads, crackers, pasta, peas, corn, winter squashes, beans, lentils, and potatoes are all starches. Whole-grain breads and crackers are better choices than those with white flour—which are highly glycemic. Bread at lunch is optional; *it cannot be saved for dinner.* Choose other starches for variety, better blood sugar maintenance, and good nutrition.

CEREALS

Hot and cold cereals can be eaten only for breakfast—and only on alternate days. Cereal should be whole-grain and unsweetened.

1–1½ cups cold cereal. Brands that are unsweetened and whole-grain:
Bran flakes
Grainfield cereals
Grape Nuts
(3 tablespoons)
Puffed rice
Puffed wheat
Shredded wheat
Wheat Chex
Wheat germ
(3 tablespoons)

1 cup cooked farina
1 cup cooked oatmeal
1 cup cooked Wheatena
1 cup Kashi

BREADS AND CRACKERS

Experiment with whole-grain breads. Rye bread is another option. If you *hate* whole-grain breads and crackers, you can use white enriched bread. But remember, it is highly glycemic and won't give the benefits of other starches. Breads should be eaten at breakfast. They are optional at lunch.

1 medium pita bread, whole-wheat
1 slice rye bread
1 slice white enriched bread (but only if you hate whole-grain bread!)
1 slice whole-grain bread
3 whole-grain crackers, such as Wasa or Finn
1 small whole-grain roll, only at lunch or dinner, limited to twice a week
2 Ry-Krisps

STARCHY CARBOHYDRATES

Starchy carbohydrates should be eaten at lunch or dinner. Women can have starchy carbohydrates on alternate days. Men can have them on a daily basis. However, if you are eating a vegetarian meal, it's mandatory to have one of these with your meal. Experiment. Try something new.

GRAINS/PASTA/RICE

Grains can be steamed, boiled, or microwaved. All grain portions are between $\frac{2}{3}$ and $\frac{3}{4}$ of a cup for men, $\frac{1}{2}$ cup for women, unless indicated, when combined with animal protein. (As part of a vegetarian meal, men can have $1\frac{1}{2}$ cups and women can have 1 cup.)

Barley
Bulgur
Couscous
Kasha
Pasta, any variety, *only at dinner*, limited to twice a week
Short- or long-grain rice, preferably brown

RICE IS NICE

Limit pasta to twice a week at the most because it is highly glycemic and too easily absorbed. You can eat your pasta for dinner, but *never* for lunch. I suggest trying something new for variety—and for better blood sugar: rice. Wild rice, black Thai rice, risotto—any of these work well with vegetables and meat, especially when simmered with garlic and onion.

In fact, according to a recent *New York Times* article, more and more people are opting for rice—with an increase of ten pounds more rice per person per year.

STARCHY VEGETABLES

Starchy vegetables can be steamed, grilled (with a brush of olive oil), or microwaved.

1 ear of corn	1 cup winter squash,
½ cup green peas	such as acorn and
1 baked potato, plain	butternut
1 cup turnips	⅔ cup yams

DRIED BEANS

These are a good source of protein for vegetarian meals. They are inexpensive and they also contain much fiber. Serving sizes are ⅔ to ¾ cup for men, ½ cup for women (when eaten with an animal protein). Portions are higher for vegetarian meals (see "Vegetarian Dining," page 83). Beans come in cans, ready to be heated up with some onions, garlic, cilantro, and other spices. You can also buy them dried. These take longer to prepare, but they do not contain any preservatives. These beans must be soaked, then rinsed carefully before being cooked. The process can take two hours. Follow the directions on the package or in a recipe book for preparing beans for cooking.

Black beans	Pinto beans
Garbanzo beans	Navy beans
Kidney beans	White beans
Lentils	

VEGETABLE CHOICES

Vegetables contain important nutrients, including calcium and other minerals, vitamins, fiber, and complex carbohydrates. Even better, they are low in calories and contain no fat, added salt, or sugar. Fresh and frozen vegetables are *always* better than canned vegetables—which *always* contain salt. Dark green and yellow vegetables, such as broccoli, spinach, and carrots, contain a wide variety of vitamins and minerals. Try to eat some of these vegetables every day. Also try to get in those vegetables high in vitamin C. They are marked with an asterisk.

Vegetables can be steamed, stir-fried, roasted, or grilled with a touch of olive oil. One-half cup cooked is the minimum amount acceptable, or 1 cup raw. You can have at least two different vegetables at mealtime, two cooked, two raw, or one cooked and one raw. A crisp salad counts as a vegetable. And remember: vegetables *must* be eaten at lunch and dinner.

Some of these vegetables can be counted toward your hard chews—if eaten at the right time and in the right amounts. (See "Hard-Chew Choices" below.) They can also be eaten in between your *scheduled* hard-chew snacks and meals. These vegetables may be munched on in between your timed snacks and as 30 to 40 percent of your meal. The most important rule? Variety. Vegetables don't have to be boring!

*Arugula
*Asparagus
 Bok choy
*Broccoli
 Cabbage (green or red)
*Cauliflower
 Celery
 Chicory
 Chinese pea pods
*Collard greens
 Cucumbers
 Daikon (Japanese radishes)
 Dandelion greens
 Eggplant (Note: Eggplant "sponges" up any oil or fat you add to it during cooking. The less the better!)
 Endive
 Escarole
 Fennel
*Green beans
 Jerusalem artichokes
 Jicama

*Kale
 Kirbys
 Kohlrabi
 Leeks
 Lettuce (Choose romaine, red-tipped, Boston—the darker green, the better. Iceberg has been found to have fewer nutrients than any other kind.)
 Mushrooms, any type
 Okra
 Onions
*Peppers, any color
 Radishes
 Scallions
*Spinach
 Summer squash
*Tomatoes (If you decide to use tomato sauce, make sure it contains no sugar or fat. And remember, tomatoes are better than sauce, and sauce is better than juice.)
 Zucchini

HARD-CHEW CHOICES

These are your control snacks, the foods you need to eat at timed intervals—the first within two hours after breakfast—to balance and maintain good blood sugar. These hard chews are the most powerful tool you have. Do not cook, shred, or chop these foods. The bigger and chunkier the package, the better. Remember, chewing moves your jaw—which stimulates the pituitary gland and gets the good-blood-sugar hormones produced at a steady, regular clip. Amounts are the same for men and women.

2	carrots	1	medium apple
10	baby carrots	1	medium pear
1	cup string beans	1	cup radishes (these
1	kirby		can be daikon,
1	cup broccoli		which are easier on
1	cup cauliflower		your stomach)
2	stalks celery	1	cup fennel bulb
1	cup red or green	4	small to medium
	cabbage		asparagus stalks

SOFT-CHEW CHOICES

Th_ _ foods are another important tool in your
_ _ _Miracle Diet plan. They must be eaten at
_ _ _ervals—the first within three hours after
_ _ _d only in the afternoon. Soft chews
_ _ higher sugar content than their hard
_ _ _terparts, and unless you are in good blood
_ _gar, they can hurt your steady climb. When
you've finished your 5-Day Miracle Diet lunch,
you need only to maintain your good blood
sugar; you do not have to stimulate your pituitary
gland. By all means enjoy a hard chew, or you can
opt for one of these instead. One note: Stay away
from overly ripe soft chews; they are too sugary.
Amounts are the same for both men and women.

1	medium peach	1	medium orange
2	small plums	1¼	cups strawberries
½	grapefruit	⅔	cup blueberries,
4	small apricots		raspberries, or
½	small		blackberries
	cantaloupe	1	medium nectarine

EMERGENCY QUICK-FIX CHOICES

These are the foods you can grab when a craving just won't stop. This can occur during your first five days of change, or when the psychological *fathead* rears its . . . well, head. The foods listed below won't add extra pounds or hurt your blood-sugar balance. They supply the sweetness, or "carbo-call," a craving wants. They are designed to hold a craving at bay until it disappears. They are quick, and they work. Amounts are the same for both men and women.

1 slice cantaloupe
¼ orange
½ unsalted pretzel
1 unsalted, unsweetened cracker
½ slice whole-grain bread

Any vegetables on the "Vegetable Choices" list
1 apple or pear (in *addition* to whatever hard chew you choose)
Herbal teas (but stay away from sweet-tasting ones!)

"EXTRAS" FOOD FOR THOUGHT

The good-blood-sugar "golden rule" is critical when it comes time to eat your "Extra." It's also important to remember that, yes, you'll feel the "hit" of your "Extra" the next day if it's a trigger food containing sugar or alcohol. So forewarned is forearmed. The next day you'll need to recover. Be extra careful in your meal and hard chew timings, in writing how you feel in your diary. In getting in extra exercise.

But for some of us the "Extra hit" can set us off. If you're a real "Sugarbaby," I suggest you stay away from sugary items (desserts *and* sweet fruits) and alcohol when you pick your "Extra." Ditto for those of you who crave carbos. Your "hit" might make you unconscious. So . . . stay away from pasta, biscuits, and bagels—if you can. Remember, these are decisions only you can make. You are in control—when you are in good blood sugar on the 5-Day Miracle Diet. Once you "own" the program, you can do whatever you want. One or two days recuperating from your "Extras" might be worth it!

There are five categories of "Extras."

- Alcohol
- Appetizer
- More elaborate main dish
- Extra starch
- Dessert

Please note: People with high cholesterol or hypertension should follow a low-fat diet, even when it comes to "Extras." Please check with your health professional before choosing your "Food You Adore."

Here are some suggestions to get those taste buds going:

Caesar salad
Shrimp cocktail
Lobster bisque
Eggplant parmigiana
Veal chop with sauce
Roast beef and gravy
Pasta with pesto sauce
A full portion of pasta
  and whatever sauce
  you want
A sandwich with all the
  fixings on a roll
Cheese on baguette
  bread
Persian melon
Tuna fish sandwich on
  a seeded roll
Glass of ice-cold
  Chardonnay
Slice of homemade
  apple pie
A chunk of Saint André
  cheese

Hot fudge sundae
A chocolate truffle
More starch or meat
Chinese dumplings
Tekka maki
Szechuan chicken with
  broccoli
A handful of walnuts
A Bloody Mary
Chicken noodle soup
Ben & Jerry's Chunky
  Monkey ice cream
Stuffed clams
Sautéed soft-shell
  crabs
Mashed potatoes
Tempura
Hamburger on a roll
Hot dog and
  sauerkraut
Banana cream pie
Chili
Frozen yogurt

In short, enjoy what you like—as long as you know the rules!

CONDIMENT CHOICES

Use this list at any time to spice up your food or to take a low-cal break.

All spices and herbs are permissible. Reduced-sodium products are always preferable—and they are mandatory if you are seeing a medical professional for any heart condition.

All mustards are okay, except honey mustard and other sweetened mustards.

No ketchup. It has too much sugar.

Use cold-pressed or virgin oil.

Vegetable and nonfat chicken broth are both fine, but watch the sodium levels.

Stick to clear or vinaigrette salad dressings. Avoid any heavy dressings such as French, Russian, blue cheese, or any honey mustards.

No nonfat salad dressings. To replace the taste of fat, they have added sugar—lots of it.

Herbal teas are fine, but they must be unsweetened and not sweet-flavored ones.

All types of water are okay, except flavored seltzer. The only flavored seltzer that won't upset your blood sugar is lemon/lime.

FAT CHOICES

Fat is fattening. But it also tastes good. And a small amount of unsaturated fats is necessary every day to supply the body with the essential fatty acids it cannot manufacture on its own. These fatty acids make for glowing skin, shiny hair, and good health.

Fat can make all the difference between deprivation and feeling great on the 5-Day Miracle Diet. I recommend monounsaturated or poly-unsaturated vegetable oils only; these are the healthiest fats for you. The fats listed below can be used sparingly in salad dressings, for sauté-ing, and brushed on vegetables before grilling and roasting. Occasionally unsalted, unsweetened butter or light mayonnaise can be substituted for the fats below. All amounts are one teaspoon. The best choices, in terms of heart health and cancer prevention, are canola oil and olive oil.

Canola oil	Safflower oil
Corn oil	Soybean oil
Olive oil	Sunflower oil
Peanut oil	

WEIGHTS AND MEASURES

In the real world you don't take a scale with you to a restaurant. Nor do you want to spend your life weighing and measuring your meals. But just to make sure you're getting the right amount, weigh your food *once* and only once, and eyeball it from then on. (If you start to gain weight, reweigh your food; it might be your portions.)

Here are some rules of thumb:

- 3 ounces of protein is about the size of a deck of cards
- 2 ounces of protein is the size of a chicken leg
- 1 ounce is around the size of a tea bag
- 2 ounces of cottage cheese is about the same size as a golf ball
- 1 medium fruit, such as an apple, is the size of a tennis ball
- 1 tablespoon is about the size of a quarter
- 1 teaspoon is about the size of a nickel

THE SAME APPLE, BUT DIFFERENT BITES

When Adam and Eve bit into the infamous apple and discovered the differences between the sexes, there was more to it than anatomy, especially when it comes to diet. There's nothing spiritual or psychological about it. It's just physical. Men are generally larger than women and are able to metabolize food more efficiently. Pure and simple, it's in their hormonal makeup to have more muscle, which burns better than fat tissue. Add the fact that women have more layers of fat for childbearing purposes (and monthly cycles that cause them to retain water), and you can see why men can eat more than women and get the same results.

The 5-Day Miracle Diet accommodates this difference between men and women:

WOMEN

Breakfast: 1–2 ounces protein and 1 starch
Lunch: 2–4 ounces protein (no starchy carbohydrates if eating them for dinner—and on alternate days only!)
Dinner: 2–4 ounces protein (no starchy carbohydrates if you ate them at lunch—and on alternate days only!)
Fat: 1–3 teaspoons
Fruit: 2 (as morning or afternoon snacks)

(In general, choose the lower allowable amounts on the food-choices lists.)

If you are over 250 pounds, add one more ounce of protein at each mealtime. Starchy carbohydrates can be eaten once every day, at either lunch or dinner. You can also add an additional fruit.

You may eat the larger portion of protein at lunch instead of dinner.

MEN

Breakfast: 2 ounces protein and 1–2 starches
Lunch: 3–4 ounces protein (starchy
carbohydrates allowed for
lunch or dinner)
Dinner: 3–6 ounces protein (starchy
carbohydrates allowed for
lunch or dinner)
Fat: 3–6 teaspoons
Fruit: 3 (as morning or afternoon snacks)

(In general choose the higher allowable amounts on the food-choices lists.)

If you are over 275 pounds, add one more ounce of protein and one more starchy carbohydrate portion at each mealtime. You can choose a fourth fruit, if you need it.

You may eat the larger portion at lunch instead of dinner.

❤ ❤ ❤ ❤ ❤ ❤ ❤ ❤ ❤ ❤

TYPICAL BREAKFAST CHOICES

(Women should choose the lower-portion amounts. Men should choose the higher-portion amounts.)

PROTEIN

You can mix and match your choices, but do not exceed the noted amounts. For example, you can have 1 slice of cheese and 1 egg.

2–3 egg whites
1 egg yolk and 2 egg whites
3–4 ounces tofu or tempeh
2–3 teaspoons peanut butter, without sugar or salt. (This is high in fat, so limit it. Avoid low-fat peanut butter—it has sugar!)
1/3–3/4 cup no-fat or 1% cottage cheese or whey cheese
2 slices no-fat cheese
2 ounces tuna or salmon, water-packed or fresh
2 ounces chicken, skinless
2 ounces fish
2 ounces hard cheese (High in fat, so limit it.)

STARCHY CARBOHYDRATES

1 slice whole-grain bread
2 rice cakes
1 slice rye bread
1 slice white enriched bread (but only if you hate whole-grain bread!)

TYPICAL LUNCH AND DINNER CHOICES

(Women should choose the lower-portion amounts. Men should choose the higher-portion amounts.)

PROTEIN

You can mix and match your choices, but do not exceed the noted amounts. For example, you can have 2 ounces tuna and 3 ounces chicken without the skin.

- 1–2 eggs
- 2 egg whites
- 2 egg whites and 1 yolk
- 1/3–3/4 cup no-fat or 1% fat cottage cheese or whey cheese
- 1–2 ounces hard cheese (no more than 60% fat)
- 2–3 slices no-fat cheese
- 3–5 ounces tuna or salmon, water-packed or fresh
- 3–5 ounces fish, any type, grilled, smoked, broiled, or poached
- 3–5 ounces chicken, without skin
- 3–5 ounces turkey, without skin, smoked or fresh
- 4–5 ounces tofu or tempeh
- 3–5 ounces Cornish hen, skinless
- 3–5 ounces shellfish, such as lobster, shrimp, or clams
- 3–5 ounces lean beef, pork, or lamb (Try to limit these higher-fat proteins. If you've been eating red meat six times a week, try to cut down to once or twice a week. If you've been eating red meat only once a week, try to cut down to once or twice a month.)

VEGETABLES

Any variety of nonstarchy vegetables, either steamed, grilled, stir-fried, or raw in a salad. Eat at least two servings of vegetables at dinner.

STARCHY CARBOHYDRATES

(At dinner *or* lunch, every day for men, alternate days for women)

1 medium baked potato
½–1 cup brown rice
½–1 cup pasta (at dinner only)
½–¾ cup corn
½–¾ cup peas
½–1 cup barley, kasha, or other grains
½–1 cup couscous
½–¾ cup beans, such as garbanzo, pinto, black, kidney, and white beans

CHAPTER 4

Give Me Five Days

If you told me five days ago that I wouldn't miss my morning roll and butter, I would have told you to get lost. Now it's "Roll and butter? What's a roll?" I can't believe it, but I don't miss it at all!
   —A fifty-four-year-old male stockbroker

Marsha would be the first to tell you. She was a mess when she first came to see me. She was twenty pounds overweight and depressed—and, at forty-one, she was nervous and worried about her health.

"I've tried everything, Adele. I want to be healthy. I want to have energy. I want to look good. But somehow, some way, I always gain the weight back."

Marsha sighed. She felt like a failure. I understood. I listened. Marsha had been heavy her whole life, just enough to make her feel self-conscious about her looks. It affected her self-image and her success. Consequently she could never sustain a relationship. Her finances were a mess; her studio apartment was impersonal, cold. She was talented and intelligent, but after college she went from one retail job to another. I nodded. There was nothing she could tell me that I hadn't heard before. I'd been there myself. I wasn't standing in judgment. I wanted to help.

And help I did. When Marsha realized that it was her body and its chemical ventriloquist that made her go on and off diets, she actually smiled. There was hope in her eyes again.

"You mean it's not all in my head?"

"Some of it is, but the bulk of your problem is a physical

103

one. It's like trying to go up a down escalator all day long with a hundred-pound pack on your back."

"Wow." Marsha clasped her hands. "Maybe. Maybe this will work."

I told Marsha what I tell everyone, and what I tell you: "Give me five days and I'll change your life."

FOOD FOR THOUGHT

You do not have an eating disorder. You have a chemical disorder.

THE DAY BEFORE

Congratulations! You've decided to start the 5-Day Miracle Diet. But before you begin, there are some things to keep in mind to enhance your success.

Timing might be everything, but we can't always control the situations in which we find ourselves. Illness, family problems, job pressure, even positive stress, such as falling in love or getting a promotion, can make us anxiously run out for cookies and milk (or champagne and caviar). We can't change the stress—but we can change the way we handle it.

Hope is a light diet, but very stimulating.
—Honoré de Balzac

There are certain stresses that we may be in a position to anticipate. A best friend's wedding. A college reunion. An important job interview. A long-awaited cruise in the Caribbean. Because we know about these events well in advance, we can plan for them. We can carefully decide what to wear, what to take—and what to eat.

That brings us to the 5-Day Miracle Diet. Why start your five days when you know you're going to a wedding or a party? At this point, what's a few more days?

So ... plan carefully. Block out a good five days in your appointment calendar (or at least an approaching empty three days). Buy a notebook to use as your food diary, or photocopy the blank food-diary page at the back of this book.

Another suggestion: Go to your supermarket the night before you begin. Better yet, visit an organic-produce stand or the newest gourmet store. Choose bright orange carrots. Plump green kirbys. Juicy red apples. Succulent pears. Treat yourself. You deserve it. You're going to change your life the very next day!

Facilitate the program by deciding what you're going to eat in the morning at the same time you're thinking about what to wear. Wrap up your hard chews so that all you have to do is put them in your bag.

DIETING THROUGH HISTORY

In Napoleonic France the waif look was "in" long before Kate Moss was even a dot on the horizon. Women got their svelte look by starving themselves, lying around on couches, and getting sick—literally. They'd wear sheer muslin in zero-degree weather and come down with pneumonia. Hey, there's nothing like a good bug to keep cravings at bay!

WHAT TO DO ON DAY ONE

Okay, it's here. You wake up and, of course, there's no
time for breakfast. Guess you'll have to wait before you
can go on your diet. No! You realize that it's a simple
matter of taking a slice of no-fat cheese and putting it on
a slice of whole-grain bread. You can eat it on the run.
Grabbing two carrots and an apple, you stuff them into
your attaché case along with your appointment book.
You did it. You're on your way.

I told Marsha to call me during the week if she ran into
any problems. Sure enough, in the middle of the morning
of her first day, the phone rang. It was Marsha. She was
tense, anxious, and thinking about food. "Help!"

I told her to take a deep breath and, as the advertise-
ment says, "Just do it!" To help handle the cravings you
might experience, "hit" on a small amount of fruit or
starch, an orange segment, or half of a pretzel. Look over
the "Quick Fix" list on page 92. All these foods will get
you over the craving without projecting bad blood sugar.
They'll get you past the danger zone for the moment.
And the good news? Each day the cravings will become a
little less.

Think about it. Your body is going through tremendous changes. You have probably never been in good
blood sugar in your entire life. We've taken away the
constant diet of "hits." You now have only little hits and
they're much more sedate than those sugary, carbo-laden
rushes you're used to. The cravings might feel intense
the first few days; you're going through a major change.
But stay with it. It takes about five days for the good
blood sugar to take hold—and then you'll feel great!

Although you might initially feel strange, your body is
getting healthy—for perhaps the very first time.

The cravings *will* go away. I promise. Just continue to write in your diary, time your meals and snacks, and wait. It gets easy.

1. "Shoot the Scale." Weigh yourself—then tuck your scale away in the closet.
2. Make the simplest meals and snacks so that you don't have to think about the diet or food. Carry your snacks with you wherever you go. Plan ahead, or you'll end up in the office cafeteria, where the bagels are calling your name.
3. Write down the ways your body is going to change in your food diary.
4. At the end of Day One, pack your food for the next day, right after dinner. It helps with your resolve to be organized and to plan ahead.
5. Planning ahead also means weighing the different foods—for the first and *only* time, so that you'll have an idea of portion size without carrying around a scale and measuring spoons!
6. Don't analyze. Don't worry about the program or how you feel. Just tell yourself it's only five days. This, too, shall pass. Just do it!

DAY ONE: SAMPLE MENU FOR WOMEN

Breakfast: (7:30)	2 ounces no-fat Cheddar cheese
	1 slice eight-grain bread
Hard-chew snack: (9:30)	10 baby carrots
Hard-chew snack: (11:30)	1 cup (healthy handful) string beans
Lunch: (12:30)	"Mock" chef's salad: Large chopped salad with 4 ounces sliced turkey as only deli meat

Sprinkle with balsamic vinegar and 2 teaspoons olive oil. Celery in salad for "tying the ribbon" on good blood sugar (GBS) 1 roll (1 ounce)

Soft- or hard-chew
snack: (3:30)   1 medium orange
Dinner: (6:00)   Chinese takeout: ½ cup brown rice with steamed vegetables and 6 ounces bean curd (tofu)

Day One comment: "I feel like I'm on another planet. Slightly dizzy. A little unfocused. But definitely proud of myself for starting!"

DAY ONE: SAMPLE MENU FOR MEN
Breakfast: (7:00)   2 ounces no-fat hard cheese
                    2 slices eight-grain bread
Hard-chew snack: (9:00)   10 baby carrots
Hard-chew snack: (11:00) 1 cup (healthy handful) string beans
Lunch: (12:30)   "Mock" chef's salad: Large chopped salad with 3 ounces sliced turkey and 1 sliced egg (and celery to "tie the bow" on GBS), with balsamic vinegar and 2 teaspoons olive oil
                    1-ounce whole-wheat roll
Soft- or hard-chew
snack: (3:30)   1 medium orange

Soft- or hard-chew snack: (6:00)	1 pear
Dinner: (7:00)	Chinese takeout: ⅔ cup brown rice with steamed vegetables, 1 teaspoon peanut oil, and 6 ounces bean curd (tofu)
Day One comment:	"Had a hard chew for my second afternoon snack. I know it doesn't matter in P.M., and I felt like a pear. Easy to follow. Since I was eating dinner at 7:00, had to have that second snack, okay. So far, so good. Only a little tempting when S. brought in the homemade cake, but hard chew took care of that."

▲ ▲ ▲ ▲ ▲ ▲ ▲ ▲ ▲

MY PLAN IS YOUR PLAN

I can tell you five hundred things to do to help you get in good blood sugar, but if I tell them to you all at once, or even spaced out over a couple of weeks, I've lost you. You'll give up. Better for me to give you ten good hints that you can do. Only ten. Or one. Or two. You'll come back for more. Then you'll own the 5-Day Miracle Diet. It will be yours. Not because I told you to do a list of things, but because you want to do them. You want to do *it*.

And I have to tell you, for me, that's the biggest high of all.

▼ ▼ ▼ ▼ ▼ ▼ ▼ ▼ ▼

DAY TWO

The alarm sounds at seven-thirty. You stretch and think about breakfast: blueberry pancakes shimmering with syrup and a rasher of bacon. You smile—then gasp. "What's happening to me? I'm thinking more about food than I did yesterday!"

You're not alone. Marsha called me the second day with the very same complaint—and so have a few thousand other clients. Remember, your body is going through incredible changes. Your chemical blood-sugar balance is going from bad to good. You're getting better. Just hold on!

If things get really tough, remember your "Quick Fix" list. Use it. That's what it's there for. You also might want to spread around some "inspiration." A Post-It on your bathroom mirror. A note taped to the door to remind you to take your chews to work . . .

WHAT TO DO ON DAY TWO

1. Use a "Quick Fix" if you need to. Go for the sugar in the slice of orange or the carbo content of a half unsalted pretzel.
2. Don't beat yourself up if you slip. This is a nonguilt program.
3. Stay busy. Do that mindless work you've been putting off in the office. Do your closets. Go to sleep early. Anything. Remember, you're almost there.
4. Keep track of your foods and emotions in your food diary.
5. Continue to keep your food simple. Prepare your hard and soft chews for the next day and store them in the refrigerator.

6. Remember your water.
7. Tell yourself that tomorrow you are going to feel better than you ever have in your entire life!

DAY TWO: SAMPLE MENU FOR WOMEN

Breakfast: (7:30)	1 bowl shredded wheat 1 cup skim milk
Hard-chew snack: (9:30)	Healthy handful of red cabbage
Hard-chew snack: (11:30)	1 apple
Lunch: (1:00)	Grilled vegetables brushed with small amount of olive oil (including uncooked hard-chew carrot to tie ribbon on good blood sugar) 4 ounces grilled shrimp 1 slice rye bread
Quick Fix: (2:30)	1 segment orange
Soft- or hard-chew snack: (4:00)	½ cantaloupe
Dinner: (7:00)	⅔ cup black beans simmered with onions, garlic, peppers, and cilantro ½ cup cooked brown rice Mixed greens with balsamic vinegar
Quick Fix: (8:30)	2 celery stalks
Day Two comment:	"Felt liberating not to weigh things anymore. But harder to stick to than yesterday. 'Quick Fixes' helped. Determined!"

DAY TWO: SAMPLE MENU FOR MEN

Breakfast: (7:30 after
exercising) Bowl of shredded
wheat
1 cup 1% milk

Hard-chew snack: (9:30) Healthy handful of red
cabbage

Hard-chew snack: (11:30) 1 apple

Lunch: (1:00) Grilled vegetables
brushed with olive oil
(including uncooked
hard-chew carrot)
4 ounces grilled shrimp
1 small roll

Soft- or hard-chew
snack: (4:00) ½ cantaloupe

Soft- or hard-chew
snack: (7:00) 1 apple

Dinner: (7:30) ⅔ cup black beans
simmered with garlic,
onions, peppers, and
cilantro
1 cup cooked brown rice
Mixed greens with
balsamic vinegar and
olive oil

Day Two comment: "Exercise helped. Still
felt cravings but
motivation strong.
For some reason, I like
a hard chew in the
afternoon. Makes me
more energetic."

WHAT TO DO ON DAY THREE

It's happened. Yes. You're beginning to feel it. The energy. The vitality. The confidence. In fact your first thought this morning wasn't about food. It was about the weather, the way the early sun hit your blinds. And there, in the corner, your treadmill. If you didn't use it yesterday, you think about using it today. Suddenly, you decide that maybe it shouldn't be a substitute closet. Suddenly, you actually think about using it!

Getting into good blood sugar takes your body anywhere from forty-eight to seventy-two hours. And when it happens, it's better than any sugar hit you ever had. By Day Three you will start to:

- Feel wonderful
- Have more energy and focus
- Begin to lose weight

As Marsha wrote in her diary for Day Three, "I feel empowered. I can't believe it. Empowered. That's exactly right."

> There is no medicine like hope, no incentive so great, and no tonic so powerful as expectation of something tomorrow.
>
> —O. S. Marden

1. Smile. You're starting to notice a real change in your attitude and your vigor.
2. Keep your food diary—and record your positive emotions.
3. Think about some exercise you might want to do when you're ready, something you might have enjoyed as a

child, such as horseback riding, or something you've wanted to do lately, such as in-line skating.

4. Before beginning your day, sit up in bed and close your eyes. Take several deep breaths. Enjoy the way your body and mind feel!

IT ALL COMES DOWN TO SHOPPING BAGS

One of my clients knows when she's about to slip: She runs out of grocery bags. "There I am, thinking about a chocolate bar or some runny Brie with crusty French bread, and sure enough, I haven't gone shopping; I don't have any grocery bags in my apartment."

When this client is in good blood sugar, she goes to the grocery store on a regular basis to pick up fresh produce and meats. She has a constant supply of grocery bags and food on hand. Sure enough, when she runs out, it's time to rethink, reevaluate, and get back on track.

DAY THREE: SAMPLE MENU FOR WOMEN

Breakfast: (8:00 after
workout on treadmill) 1 slice whole-grain
bread
2 teaspoons
unsweetened peanut
butter
Hard-chew snack: (10:00) 10 baby carrots
Lunch: (12:00) ½ cup couscous
1 broiled lamb chop
Mixed salad (with
chunks of whole
radishes) drizzled with

balsamic vinegar and
2 teaspoons oil
Steamed vegetables
1 bottle San Pellegrino

Soft- or hard-chew
　　　snack: (3:00) 1¼ cups strawberries
Soft- or hard-chew
　　　snack: (6:00) 1 apple
　　Dinner: (7:00) *Vegetarian meal:*
1 bowl lentil soup
1 large plate steamed
mixed vegetables mixed
with 1 teaspoon oil
Perrier and lime

Day Three comment: "It's beginning. I can
feel it. It's like I lost a
deadweight or an extra-
heavy suitcase. I'm free!
Dare I say my cravings
are gone?"

DAY THREE: SAMPLE MENU FOR MEN

　　Breakfast: (7:30
after exercising) 2 slices whole-grain
bread
1–1½ tablespoons
unsweetened peanut
butter
Hard-chew snack: (9:30) 10 baby carrots
Hard-chew snack: (11:00) 1 apple
　　Lunch: (12:30) ¾ cup couscous
1 medium broiled lamb
chop
Steamed zucchini
Mixed green salad

	(containing 1 cup raw broccoli chunks) with 1 tablespoon of vinaigrette dressing

Soft- or hard-chew
snack: (3:00) 1¼ cups strawberries
Quick Fix: (4:15) ½ unsalted pretzel
Dinner: (6:00) *Vegetarian meal:*
1 bowl lentil soup
1 large plate steamed
mixed vegetables
1 slice whole-grain bread
Large bottle mineral
water

Day Three comment: "For some reason it was
harder today than it
was yesterday! I actually
needed a 'Quick Fix.'
Listening to my body.
It's changing. I know this
will pass. Everything
tastes better—even
water."

"TAKE IT BACK"

While the 5-Day Miracle Diet might not actually encourage relapses, it doesn't discourage them, either. Relapses make you human. You can learn from them. Call it practice. You'll be amazed at the confidence you'll feel when you get back on track. You did it!

After a few weeks on the 5-Day Miracle Diet, you will go longer and longer without shaking up your good blood sugar. And when those extra-indulgent times occur, you'll recover it very quickly. Why? Because you'll love the way you feel when you're in good blood sugar and you'll want to get back—fast.

WHAT TO DO ON DAY FOUR

Yes, you're getting the rhythm. Your feet feel lighter. You walk right by the French bakery and don't even notice the croissants in the window. But wait. As the light on the street corner changes, you panic. It's the weekend! Will this good feeling last? Will the cravings stay quiet? But it's only Saturday morning and you have nothing planned. . . .

What you need are some well-attuned strategies to get you through the next two days. It's well past time to be nice to yourself with some nonfood rewards. Here are some suggestions I gave Marsha:

- Go to a movie you've been dying to see—and smile smugly at the line of people waiting for greasy, fatty popcorn
- Call a friend you haven't spoken to in a while
- Read a good thriller or a great romance

- Take that kick-boxing class you've been meaning to sign up for at the gym
- Get a manicure and a pedicure
- Go for a massage
- Shop till you drop—or simply browse through the mall
- Play a game of tennis
- Take a walk
- Start an impromptu basketball game with the neighbors
- Visit a museum
- Join a baseball game in the park

1. Notice how good you're beginning to feel.
2. Keep telling yourself you're only one day away from balanced blood sugar—and the end of your cravings!
3. Take time out to realize how good you feel about yourself. You're not even hungry!
4. Try on a skirt or a pair of pants that were a little too tight around the waist one week ago.
5. Continue to record your feelings and your foods in your diary.

Eating an artichoke is like getting to know someone really well.

—Willi Hastings

DAY FOUR: SAMPLE MENU FOR WOMEN

Breakfast: (7:30) 2 slices turkey
1 slice eight-grain bread

Hard-chew snack: (9:30) 2 stalks celery

Hard-chew snack: (11:30) 1 apple

Lunch: (12:30) 1 can tuna, packed in spring water, with

<table>
<tr><td></td><td>lettuce, tomato, and mustard
Salad (with uncooked carrot slices) and
1 teaspoon vinaigrette dressing
1 slice rye bread</td></tr>
<tr><td>Soft- or hard-chew snack: (3:30)</td><td>2 tangerines</td></tr>
<tr><td>Dinner: (6:00)</td><td>Chinese takeout:
Steamed vegetables, chicken, and brown rice</td></tr>
<tr><td>Day Four comment:</td><td>"I can't believe it. A weekend and I'm up early—because I want to be! Feel great. Went to gym. Met a friend for lunch. Saw a movie and didn't crave popcorn. In fact didn't even need my 'Quick Fix.' Just my bottle of water."</td></tr>
</table>

DAY FOUR: SAMPLE MENU FOR MEN

Breakfast: (8:30)	2 slices turkey 1 slice eight-grain bread
Hard-chew snack: (10:30)	2 stalks celery
Lunch: (12:30)	One hamburger with lettuce, tomato, and mustard on pita bread Salad (with carrot strips) and vinaigrette dressing
Soft- or hard-chew snack: (3:30)	1 apple

Dinner: (6:00)   Chinese takeout:
                  Steamed vegetables,
                  scallops and shrimp,
                  brown rice
Day Four comment: "Feel great! I can't
                  believe it. The best
                  night's sleep I've had
                  in years. Getting used to
                  water. Didn't even wake
                  up in the middle of the
                  night to go to bathroom.
                  My skin's better. Skin! I
                  can't believe I'm even
                  looking at my skin!
                  My whole outlook is
                  changing. I even spent
                  the day walking, just
                  walking, around the
                  city."

WHAT TO DO ON DAY FIVE

I'll never forget Marsha's face when she came back to my office. Her skin glowed. Her complexion was smooth. She had lost that bloated look.

"I didn't really believe you five days ago. I couldn't imagine feeling this good—without feeling deprived." Marsha smiled.

She got up to "shoot the scale"—and she'd lost three pounds.

As happy as that made her, Marsha almost shrugged it off. The confidence she had was worth much more than a few pounds. Losing that cloud of despair was a whole lot better than losing three pounds.

The same will happen to you. Just as it has for thousands of my other clients.

▲   ▲   ▲   ▲   ▲   ▲   ▲   ▲   ▲

FACE THE FOOD

Believe it or not, when you're in good blood sugar, you simply don't think about food. As I've often said to my clients, I would no sooner go into my favorite restaurant in low blood sugar than I would go in stark naked!

▼   ▼   ▼   ▼   ▼   ▼   ▼   ▼   ▼

1. Continue to write in your food diary.
2. It's time now to weigh yourself once again. Jot down how much you've lost during these past five days.
3. Start to plan the next week—and when you want to eat the "Food You Adore." Remember, now that you are in good blood sugar, you are in control. *You* can choose what you want to eat—rather than being controlled by your blood-sugar ventriloquist. You can eat anything you want as an "Extra." *You* control your body—not the other way around. Just don't forget Adele Puhn's Four Rules of Selectivity (see pages 57–58).
4. Treat yourself to a special nonfood reward. A movie. A ticket to a tennis match. An hour of private time away from the kids. You deserve it!
5. Congratulate yourself. You did it. You've incorporated the 5-Day Miracle Diet into your life. You now "own" the diet—and no one can ever take it away from you.

WHAT'S BRUNCH?

Yes, I know. It's that Sunday ritual that combines breakfast and lunch—and makes you sleepy and utterly useless for the rest of the day! The 5-Day Miracle Diet does not know the word *brunch*. You simply eat your breakfast when you wake up, then consider that Sunday buffet your lunch. This way you'll maintain that good GBS feeling the whole day through.

DAY FIVE: SAMPLE WEEKEND MENU FOR WOMEN

Breakfast: (10:30)	Bowl of puffed wheat 1 cup skim milk
Lunch: (12:30)	Grilled vegetables, including 1 uncooked carrot and 1 teaspoon oil 3 ounces poached salmon
Hard-chew snack: (2:30)	1 apple
Soft- or hard-chew snack: (4:30)	10 baby carrots
Soft- or hard-chew snack: (6:30)	Handful of string beans
Dinner: (7:30)	1½ cups pasta with tomato and basil sauce Huge salad with oil and vinegar ½ cup blueberries for dessert 1 bottle San Pellegrino
Day Five comment:	"Actually went to the gym today. On a Sunday! It feels easy now. As if I always did it. Slept late— and still kept with plan.

> Guess I 'own' it now—
> and no one, only myself,
> can take it away!"

DAY FIVE: SAMPLE WEEKEND MENU FOR MEN

Breakfast: (10:30)	Bowl of puffed wheat 1 cup 1% milk
Lunch: (12:30)	1 slice pizza Mixed salad with balsamic vinegar and some uncooked celery
Hard-chew snack: (2:30)	1 apple
Soft- or hard-chew snack: (4:30)	1 pear
Soft- or hard-chew snack: (6:30)	2 carrots
Soft- or hard-chew snack: (7:30)	Handful of cauliflower florettes
Dinner: (8:00)	Pasta primavera made with a little olive oil Huge salad with balsamic vinegar, olive oil, and fresh oregano 1 cup raspberries espresso 1 bottle San Pellegrino with lime
Day Five comment:	"Wow . . . Wow . . . Yeah, wow. Slept late, had pizza, went to gym, went out for dinner. Even had dessert. You call this a diet? I call it a dream come true."

5-DAY MIRACLE DIET SECRETS

- Stay *totally* away from alcohol and sugar in the beginning. You're still not in sustained good blood sugar and you're vulnerable to a craving "hit." You need five uninterrupted days so that you will know exactly what good blood sugar feels like. Tough it out. Otherwise you'll never know how good you can feel!
- Wait until your second week to eat the "Foods You Adore." Remember the number-one Adele Puhn Rule of Selectivity. You *must* be in good blood sugar. Otherwise you'll eat or drink too much and it will be harder to get back on track.
- If there are any social events that you must go to, it doesn't mean you have to forget your diet program. Go easy on yourself. If you're going out to dinner, just try not ordering a drink. That's it. Simply forget the glass of wine—or the dessert. And eat everything else in between that feels important to you.
- Another social tip: If a pending social event makes you nervous, eat your snacks and dinner before venturing out. You'll be less tempted to eat. And always eat a quick hard chew before your arrival. When you are more accustomed to the program and in good chemistry, you'll feel confident enough to wait and eat at the party. You won't give it another thought—except for the sense of well-being and pleasant fullness you'll feel!
- Think spice during your first five days. In addition to your "Quick Fix" list, try adding spice to your life with veggies dipped in salsa, tuna mixed with mustard. Salads livened up with dried spice mixes, such as Mrs. Dash. Your taste buds will get a "kick"—and that craving will disappear.

As a trimmer, more confident Marsha said at the end of her five days, "So this is what being in good blood sugar is. Unbelievable. It's a whole other dimension. I've never felt so amazing in my entire life. Why did I wait so long!!!"

Happily the waiting is over for Marsha—and for you. You are ready to change your life, your outlook, and the way you look and feel.

Good luck with your five days. In less than a week you, too, will lose 75 percent of the reason you crave certain foods. And once your body is in good blood sugar, we'll go on to the next component of the 5-Day Miracle Diet: the other 25 percent that I call the *fathead*. It's all in the next chapter.

THE 5-DAY MIRACLE MANTRA

Say this over and over again: There is no such thing as guilt on the 5-Day Miracle Diet. There is no cheating. You're simply eating more or eating less.

CHAPTER 5

The Powerful *Fathead:* The Emotional Games People Play

My issues weigh more than all the weight I've lost and gained over the years.
—A twenty-nine-year-old client and a manager of a large retail store

Congratulations! You've finished your five days of biochemical change and your body feels wonderful! Energy, confidence—all this and more are yours.

But wait a minute. What about the cookie you ate at your mother's last night because she didn't like your haircut and you suddenly felt anxious? Or the champagne you wanted desperately to drink at the wedding when you saw your ex with another (younger) beau and the pain hit you like a ton of bricks? If the entire reason we eat and crave certain foods were *all* biochemical, my book would end here. However, there is that other 25 percent, that ubiquitous mind "saboteur" I call the *fathead,* the emotional underpinnings that can sabotage any diet plan.

The *fathead* can rear its, um, head, under almost any condition or situation. The psychological, emotional reasons you reach for food can be as unique as you yourself are from everybody else. Even in good blood sugar the *fathead* is ready to tempt you away from your best-laid plans. An argument with your boss. Rejection. Too many deadlines. Stress in any shape or form—from receiving a promotion or planning a wedding to divorce and death.

All these can make you blank out and reach for food for that instant hug, that momentary numbness, that soft, mindless feeling that keeps anxiety or depression at bay.

There's only one trouble: The "hit" is over almost as soon as it began. The thoughts come back, the pain, the worry, the hurt—and, thanks to the physiological repercussions of low blood sugar, much stronger than before. Add the guilt and anger you feel from blanking out, and you have that walk up the down escalator with a pack on your back all over again.

It doesn't have to be this way. You can recognize the *fathead*'s welcome mat and you can learn the ways to close the door in its face—or, even if you've invited it in for (fattening) dinner, you can learn techniques to recover . . . fast.

▲ ▲ ▲ ▲ ▲ ▲ ▲ ▲ ▲

Life is the sacred mystery singing to itself, dancing to its drum, telling tales, improvising, playing.

—Manitonquat

▼ ▼ ▼ ▼ ▼ ▼ ▼ ▼ ▼

FOOD IS LOVE / FOOD IS HATE

As the opening credits appeared on the onetime hit series *Rhoda*, her voice was heard describing who she was and where she came from in a scant minute or two. The most defining statement? "Food was the first thing that loved me back."

We all laughed. We all identified. Even in today's popular culture, a world where our relationship with food is given the label *eating disorder*, we turn to sweet desserts or bread and butter or chocolate morsels to assuage our worries/fears/hurt/pain—take your pick. We eat our emotions instead of feeling them. But, as with any quick fix, the emotions continue to haunt us, coming back stronger than ever—thanks to our biochemistry trigger.

Food is love. And below the surface it is also hate— the profound self-loathing that enables us to focus on how "fat, ugly, disgusting, and depressed" we feel so that we don't have to look at our *own* behaviors, our *own* role in the reason we were rejected, or why we failed, or why we didn't fulfill our dreams.

Food is love. Go past the cliché and think about what those words mean. Food is love. How sad. How profound. How devious!

We can get past the *fathead*. I know. I have—as have thousands of my clients. And this chapter will help you learn not only how to identify your own particular *fatheads*—but also how to deal with them successfully.

THE BEAUTIFUL TEACHER AND THE SIZE-SIX SKIRT

Her name was Donna. You would never consider her obese, just slightly overweight. But Donna felt big, ugly. She was beautiful, but she didn't see it. She just saw the twenty pounds of extra fat that had been with her since grade school.

"I've tried everything. Diet pills. No-fat, no-carbohydrate diets. Liquid diets. Group-support diets. Even injections of animal placenta. Oh, sure, I always lost weight—until the need to eat reared its ugly (fat) head again. Food called to me. It sang to me. It rang inside my very soul."

Donna always gained weight—until she came to me. "You were my last-ditch effort, Adele," she told me, sitting in a chair in my office. "If you told me I could never eat a piece of chocolate cake again, I would have gotten up, said thanks a lot, and never come back."

But as all of you now know, I never said that. I told her about the physiological reasons why she ate. I told her about my diet plan—and how, after five days, I *insisted* she eat something she adores once or twice a week: from a Caesar salad to, yes, double-rich, double-fudge chocolate cake.

Donna liked the idea that much of the reason she ate was biochemical. She tried my five-day "start-up" and soon she was in good blood sugar, and feeling stronger and more energetic than ever. She'd go to her job as a sixth-grade teacher and come home without flinging herself on her sofa. She'd spend quality time with her son, do some errands, and enjoy a few hours with her husband before going to sleep.

She did great. She lost the thirty-five pounds she'd gained when she was pregnant. But suddenly the twenty pounds she could never lose reared its ugly head. "Twenty pounds," her fat seemed to whisper. "Twenty pounds." True, thanks to her balanced chemistry, Donna had a new lease on life. However, the strength she felt, the genuinely good feelings she had about herself and her life, made her nervous. Change always brings its own form of stress.

"Twenty pounds," her *fathead* said.

As it happened, she came to me the following week knowing full well she had gained weight. "I don't even want to get on the scale," she said. We "shot the scale," and sure enough, Donna had gained three pounds. "Do you think the hormonal changes of menopause can make you gain weight?" she asked me.

I nodded, but I wasn't sure if this was her issue. I glanced at Donna's food diary, and sure enough, there was plenty of evidence staring at me in black and white, such as the cookies eaten one afternoon, the ice cream consumed less than forty-eight hours later. She was teasing herself, never getting back into good blood sugar.

"Sure, Donna, hormonal changes can influence your weight, but only on a minor level. I think there's something else going on."

Donna listened. She wanted to hear what I had to say—although she didn't expect my next question, a seeming non sequitur.

"What's your relationship with your mother like, Donna?"

Donna sniffed. She nudged around in her seat. "My relationship?" she stuttered. "Well, I guess it's okay. My mom is beautiful. Really beautiful. And thin."

It was as if an 8mm home movie had flashed through her mind. Suddenly the memories, the images of the past, came pouring out. She told me stories over the next few weeks, all with the unconscious message given by her mother: "Don't compete with me. Never compete. If you try to be beautiful, too, you'll lose my love." Like the time her mother had a new skirt sitting on her bed when the new thin Donna came to visit. It was a size-six black linen. Her mother's comment? "I'd let you try it on, but I don't want you to stretch it."

Another incident: When Donna was a teenager, one night during dinner her mother said, "You'd be so pretty, Donna, if you only lost some weight." The dinner? Pasta. A vegetable cream casserole. Ice cream for dessert.

And from the very recent past, at an old, close friend's engagement party, in fact: Donna, looking and feeling thin and gorgeous, wore a slinky sequined dress to the party. For the first time in her life she really wanted to laugh and make merry. She wanted to have a fabulous time. Donna's friend was breathtaking in a raw silk Armani. Unfortunately, due to last-minute, stress-inducing emergencies, her friend had gained a few pounds prior to the party. No one could ever notice the three or four pounds, but Donna's friend, nervous, excited, and incidentally in terrible blood sugar, was feeling the weight of every single pound. She looked at the smiling Donna and felt a pang of jealousy. She couldn't help it. She blurted out, "You know, you're beginning to look just like your mother. You're even acting like her." Donna binged at the engagement party—and didn't stop for three whole days.

The moral of these stories? Donna loved her mother too much to compete. To her, food was a way to keep competition at bay—and love in her mother's heart. Much better to eat that cake than lose her mother's love. Much better to grab that cookie than admit the feelings of anger toward those you love. "Yeah, my mother was beautiful. Now, don't get me wrong, she was a great mom, nurturing and kind, but, well, okay. Okay. I never wanted to be too beautiful. I didn't want to compete with my mother. I always felt guilty."

The message was unconsciously ingrained in Donna at an early age: "Mother is to be the beauty. Not me. I have to be fat . . . and ugly."

And, for her part, Donna's mother unconsciously seduced Donna with food to keep Donna fat—and herself the beauty. She used the push-pull of food to seduce. "Eat more dessert." "You know you love my macaroni salad." "Try these pastries from the new bakery down the street." And at the same time she'd say, "Don't eat that, you're trying to lose weight," and "You can't wear my clothes, you're too fat."

And the worst part: Neither Donna nor her mother was aware of the dynamics going on. Indeed Donna's mother would be absolutely horrified to know that she'd been unconsciously undermining Donna's desire to be thin— and, on a deeper level, to feel good about herself.

MOTHER LODE

No, I'm not picking on mothers. After all, I'm one myself! But the facts of life remain: The mother is usually the nurturer. From the moment you were born, it was your mother who took care of you. When you cried, she determined if you were hungry. She would offer her breast or a bottle. She would hold you in her arms and rock you.

Your mother, the nurturer, supplied the food—even before you were born. It's no wonder that we can skip the "middlewoman" and call food a nurturer—and at the same time develop complex feelings about our mother.

Food is more than sustenance. It is more than sensual joy. It is more than contentment. Food is a powerful weapon, so powerful, in fact, that it can undo the physiological work you've done.

But there is an escape clause. It's called choice.

And in that choice is the defeat of the *fathead*.

SABOTAGE: THE FERTILE SOIL FOR FATHEADS TO GROW . . . FAT

Once your body is in good blood sugar, you can look at the "real you" without fear, without repulsion, without the negative self-image that comes part and parcel with low blood sugar. There are many reasons why your best-laid plans can go astray. The *fathead* takes on many guises. There are the following:

Psychological Factors, or "I Don't Deserve . . ."

Self-sabotage is one of the most common *fathead* issues. After all, there are reasons why you gained weight—and why you haven't taken it off. Be it fear of sexuality, fear of change, fear of the unknown, or simply fear of discovering what is really bothering you, it's a powerful motivation to stay heavy, one that can sabotage the best-laid biochemical plans.

EMOTIONAL HUNGER AND THE APPROPRIATE "FOOD"

Emotional Hunger	Emotional Food
Bored	Rent a movie.
Angry	Write down your rage (privately!).
Lonely	Call a friend—and get a pet!
Tired	Take a hot bath with aromatherapy.
Tense	Take a walk or a hot bath.
Rejected	Go to a museum. Plan an event.
Frustrated	Get caught up in a good book.

Old Behaviors and Habits, or "The First Thing I Do When I Go to My Mother's House Is Open the Refrigerator Door"

Whether it's an ice-cream pop and a few pages of a book before you go to sleep or orange juice first thing in the morning, old habits die hard. We're used to them. They're comfortable. Like old shoes. Like the weight you've never taken off . . .

Eating Your Feelings Instead of Feeling Them, or "I Hate Myself"

Raw emotion. It's difficult to feel. The pain. The anger. Sometimes you're afraid if you allow yourself to feel the anger or the disappointment, you'll go crazy—or you'll go out and kill someone. Much better to eat that chocolate. Much nicer to have second helpings of the Chicken Kiev. Much more appropriate to order dessert. As one of my clients told me, "When I eat chocolate, it has everything to do with feelings. I don't like to have feelings. Chocolate tastes good as opposed to the bitter taste of reality."

But none of these things, even if eaten with a group of friends you love or in bed under a comforter watching an old movie or even on a date with someone who shows promise, can take the place of what you really need. A hug. Reassurance. Telling someone off. Saying "I hate you!" Love. Oh, yes, love.

Early Family Roles, or "I Was, I Am, I Always Will Be the Caregiver in My Home"

Pioneers in family therapy have always maintained that each person has a role, a part to play, that is unconsciously assigned to keep the family unit in balance. Perhaps you were the one who always made everyone feel better, who took care of your brothers and sisters— and, on a deeper level, your parents—and never rebelled. Maybe you were the family clown who always tried to keep everyone's spirit up. Maybe you were the strong one. Perhaps you were the one who had to put up a good front so that everyone would feel good. Whatever your role, you didn't get what you needed, pure and simple. You never vocalized what you needed. Nobody seemed to care. You were—and remain—the victim, afraid to make a move or say the wrong thing. It doesn't matter. Whatever your role, whatever your feelings, the outcome was, and is, the same: overeating. You ate food instead of feeling your emotions, something you learned at birth: "Shhh. Don't cry. Here's more formula . . . more juice . . . a Gummi Bear."

This condition is one of being "emotionally starved." Instead of feeding that emotion, you eat physical food and gain weight. You long for what you really need, but you eat a piece of chocolate instead. The result? More overeating because the chocolate will never quite cut it. You'll never be filled because you're using food to feed an emotional need. It's like using an air conditioner to keep a room warm. It simply won't work.

FOOD—THE WEAPON OF CHOICE

Some people use guns to hurt themselves. Still others will use cigarettes or alcohol to slowly do themselves in. But "food sensualists" use food. It tastes good and you can pretend that it's not harming you. All those nasty emotions can drown in a pile of whipped cream as you "go blank" and eat. And food can also provide a double whammy. Not only can overeating hurt you, but it can hurt the ones you love. They can get angry or upset with you and bingo: You can start eating again because you are so, dare I say it, angry at them! (And at yourself!) I'd say that food is not only a weapon of choice, it's a very potent one indeed.

Other People's Food, or "Just One Bite, Please, It Took Me All Afternoon"

Picture this scenario: You and your significant other are invited to a close friend's house for dinner. It's your birthday and he's cooked up an elaborate feast. He knows you're trying to lose weight (after all, the entire world knows you're trying to lose weight), but hey, it's your birthday and all rules are suspended. Lobster bisque. Baked Brie. Soft-shell crabs sautéed in oil and garlic. Salad vinaigrette with olives and croutons. And to top it off: chocolate soufflé. How can you refuse? Look how hard he worked—just for you! But there's one fatal flaw in your friend's plan: He neglected to ask you if *your* rules were suspended on your birthday. Maybe it was done on purpose. . . .

Then there's Charlotte, the client whose office was right next door to a colleague who brought piping-hot muffins in to work every day. She knew Charlotte was on a diet; she'd once asked her what those bags of raw veggies on her desk were all about. Nonetheless every day she'd stand in Charlotte's doorway, muffin box in hand, and say, "Muffin? I purposely got those lemon poppy ones you love." And equally as predictable, Charlotte would say, "Thanks, how thoughtful!" She'd promptly pick out a muffin—and ruin all the good work she'd done over the weekend or the night before. Spending a few sessions on her *fathead* issues changed all that. The next time the "muffin lady" came to the door, Charlotte smiled and said, "Thanks. It is so nice of you. But I'm just not hungry." She kept saying "Thanks, but no thanks," and the "muffin lady" finally got the hint. Unfortunately she not only stopped offering muffins, she stopped talking to Charlotte completely. Perhaps she felt rejected; perhaps she hadn't been conscious of her aggressive actions and was shocked; perhaps she was embarrassed. Whatever. It happens. You may lose some "friends" when you lose weight. But as one of my clients said, "Makes you wonder how good a friend they were to begin with!"

TRUE-LIFE ADVENTURES

I'll never forget when Susan, one of my successful clients, came back from a trip to Canada. She
had married a Canadian and she'd gone to visit
his relatives. They hadn't seen her for a year—
during which time she'd lost over thirty pounds,
thanks to the 5-Day Miracle Diet. The last time
the relatives had seen her, they were cordial,
nothing more. But now she had suddenly become the best mother, the best wife, the best
daughter-in-law in life. Her comment? "I can't
believe they defined me by the way I look. I'm
still the same person, only I'm not afraid to say,
hey, I'm angry at your stereotyping!"

DIETING THROUGH HISTORY

Dieting for women in the Middle Ages was not
vanity. It was survival. Since they were as much
property as a castle or a horse, the only way they
could control their lives was with food. If they
starved themselves, they wouldn't have to marry a
man they didn't love. They could look ugly—and
embarrass their families. They could rebel and
choose a life not dictated by the nursery or the
kitchen. They could become women of "independent means," healers, nuns, and educators.

WHAT ARE YOUR *FATHEAD* FACTORS?

These four arenas make up the *fathead* landscape. But, in
reality, the psychological reasons for eating go deep,
very deep, sometimes to places you have never contem-
plated. It might only be a mere 25 percent of the reason

you eat, but like the small word *if*, it packs a big, *big* meaning.

To help you conquer your particular brand of *fathead*, you first have to identify it. Take a few moments to take this quiz. Answer each statement *true* or *false*. And remember, be honest! No one needs to see this but you.

Part 1A: Eating Your Feelings—Thoughts

1. After I've overeaten, I look in the mirror and feel repulsed.
2. When I'm feeling low, I can't stand to look in the mirror, period.
3. I hate myself.
4. I have no confidence. My self-esteem is at an all-time low. Losing ten pounds is the only answer.
5. I hate parties. When I go to a party, I feel that I and my fat stand out.
6. When I walk down the street, I think everyone's looking at my fat—and thinking I'm lazy or undisciplined or slothful or even stupid!
7. They're probably right.
8. I have a hard time expressing my anger.
9. I tell people off all the time—in my mind.
10. I say "I'm sorry" a lot, even when I don't mean it.
11. I need a lot of reassurance.
12. I'm insecure and I don't trust people.
13. When people tell me I'm pretty, I don't believe them.
14. Deep inside myself I know that if I was a better person, I'd be able to lose weight!
15. I won't go to the beach. Heaven forbid someone sees my thighs!
16. One thing I know for sure: Fat people are *not* happy.
17. There are many things I don't do because I feel self-conscious about my weight.

18. My emotions frighten me.
19. I get scared when I start to care for someone.
20. I always feel bad after I've strayed from my diet.
21. I think of food as "good" and "bad"—and so do my friends.
22. I feel most of my friends are thinner than me—even when they're not.
23. I love to eat. Always have.

Count the number of "trues" you have. Jot the number down and go on to part 1B.

Part 1B: Eating Your Feelings—Behaviors and Activities

24. I have an overwhelming desire to eat.
25. When I'm out in public, I eat in "approved" ways: fruit for dessert, no fried foods, salad with dressing on the side. But when I come home, watch out! I head right for the refrigerator.
26. When I've had a bad day at work, all I can think about is going home and curling up with . . . my favorite food.
27. When I'm aggravated, I can eat a whole bag of chips or cookies without even being aware of how much I've gobbled up—and within minutes!
28. It's impossible to be at a bar and not have at least one drink.
29. Celebrations mean food to me. A promotion, an engagement, a clean bill of health—what better way to celebrate than going out to dinner . . . and eating!
30. I wonder what the hidden agenda is behind the compliment "You look great!" Those three words make me hungry!
31. My mother's voice is like my conscience. I hear her

"you should do that, you should eat this" so much
that I can't wait to grab a cookie.

32. There are some friends I have whom I call my eating
pals. We can't get together without eating. Just seeing them makes me want to eat!

*Count the number of "trues" you have in this section and
add that number to what you got in part 1A. Calculate
the total for parts 1A and 1B and jot it down with the
words "Eating Your Feelings."*

Part 2: Other People's Food

33. I have trouble sticking to my diet in restaurants.

34. There are a lot of *should*s in my vocabulary—most
of which I ignore when I'm dining out with friends.

35. I just have to look at a buffet table and I tell myself,
"I'll diet tomorrow."

36. If a friend or family member tells me something is
homemade, I succumb.

37. "Just take one bite" is my password to eating three
portions.

38. I think that some of my friends liked me better fat.
They were nicer to me.

39. One of my friends always orders something fattening
in a restaurant. He always tells me to take a bite—
and doesn't eat much of the food himself!

40. When a waiter brings over an entrée that is obviously
laden with sauce, I don't ask him to take it back—
even when I specifically ordered it with sauce on the
side.

41. There's nothing more difficult than going out to dinner with my friends. I feel I have to eat and drink till
I drop!

42. When I make dinner for family or friends, it's never

    low-fat. I always use it as an excuse to make fatten-
ing foods I adore.

43. I always wait to see what everyone else is ordering
before I make my (usually fattening) choice.

44. Weddings, bar mitzvahs, confirmations—they're all
excuses to eat!

45. My friends are always making comments about my
diet, charting my progress and discussing it.

46. I'm afraid of what people will think if I don't eat
what they've cooked. I don't want to hurt their
feelings.

47. I don't know how to answer the popular question
"How much more do you want to lose?"

*Count the total number of "trues" you have in part 2 and jot
it down with the words "Other People's Food" next to it.*

Part 3: Family Feuds

48. Whenever my father and I get together, we always
seem to fight.

49. I get a lot of mixed messages from my mother. She's
always telling me to diet—as she puts another portion of pie on my plate!

50. My father was always very controlling.

51. My parents expected me to be perfect—and I always
felt I failed.

52. I was never hugged as a child.

53. I had a large family and I always felt I had to rush to
the table so that there would be something left for me
to eat!

54. My parents are always comparing me to my sib-
ling—who is thin.

55. I get embarrassed when my father tells me how
pretty I am and how I'm growing up.

56. My spouse is always telling me to lose weight—and it gets on my nerves!
57. As soon as I start to lose weight, my spouse gets jealous of anyone who even glances my way.
58. My mother dresses more youthful and sexier than me.
59. Family functions are the worst. Even if I'm in fabulous blood sugar, I'll go to my mother's house or my aunt's or wherever and my resolve . . . dissolves.
60. I never felt loved in my family.
61. I sense my parents' disapproval—even though they are long gone.
62. We never expressed our feelings in our house.
63. My parents fought almost every night.
64. I was an abused child.

Count the total number of "trues" you have in part 3 and jot it down with the words "Family Feuds" next to it.

Part 4: The Comfort Zone

65. Whenever I felt rejected or sad, my mother always made me my favorite (fattening) food for dinner.
66. I never felt closer to my family than on Sunday afternoons, watching the game on TV, and snacking, snacking, snacking.
67. Going out to dinner was a family ritual—and I miss it.
68. I can't get to sleep unless I've had some ice cream in bed.
69. There's no such thing as breakfast without orange juice.
70. I eat the same breakfast every day: a muffin and coffee.
71. I never say no when a colleague offers me food.
72. Lunch is always a sandwich at my desk.

73. Vegetables were never part of my routine.
74. I can't imagine bread without butter.
75. I don't like fish. I'm a meat-and-potatoes person.
76. I can't watch television without snacking.
77. I can't read without some food nearby.
78. I love reading the Sunday papers, a cup of coffee nearby . . . and a bagel.
79. Don't even speak to me until I've had two cups of coffee.
80. The people who work at the cafeteria know exactly what I want. They even have the hamburger ready for me when I come in.
81. I always went with my friends to the local hamburger hangout after school. A burger and fries was a staple in those days. Still is, sometimes.
82. I always believed in "feeding a cold"—or any illness, for that matter.

Count the total number of "trues" you have for part 4 and jot it down with the words "The Comfort Zone" next to it.

YOUR *FATHEAD* FOOD SCORE—AND WHAT IT MEANS

Look at the totals you have for the four different categories. See which one has the most "trues" and read the corresponding section below. If you happen to have a tie or totals that are very close, it means that your *fathead* issues involve more than one arena.

• If you had more "trues" in the statements under "Eating Your Feelings—Thoughts" and "Eating Your Feelings—Behaviors and Activities," your *fathead* issues have much to do with the way you cope. Most likely your *fathead* is an issue of low self-esteem—which goes back a long way. The emotions you feel—and hide—are the same ones you felt in your crib, on the school playground, in middle-school English class, at the prom. It's just the situations themselves that have changed—and perhaps the food you overeat to compensate for them. (Instead of a bottle or a peanut butter and jelly sandwich, it's Scotch and water or a bag of chips.) The fact is, your *fathead* would rather hide its head in a bowl of bouillabaisse than have you face your emotions.

- If you had more "trues" in the statements under "Other People's Food," your *fathead* issues most likely deal with insecurities—and the need to please others.
- If you had more "trues" in the statements under "Family Feuds," your *fathead* issues go down deep and long ago, to the relationships you had with your parents and, most likely, your mother, because she was the nurturer, supplying your food from the moment of birth.
- If you had more "trues" in the statements under "The Comfort Zone," your *fathead* issues are based on old habits and comfortable routines. Most likely you were raised to use food to assuage your feelings, to make you feel less nervous and more secure. Eating was probably a close family event and all your good times were associated with food.

THE ZOMBIE LAWYER

We used to joke about Jack being a zombie. No, he wasn't a weirdo. He didn't even watch science fiction movies. Jack was—and continues to be—a successful client of mine for over three years. He's lost over one hundred pounds and he's kept it off.

Now he talks about good blood sugar and timed snacks as if it were second nature. But it wasn't always that easy. Once Jack got into good blood sugar (or GBS) on my diet plan, his *fathead* took over. He was feeling great; he had a tremendous amount of energy; he lost his cravings.

But for three weeks in a row he couldn't lose weight. We began to examine what was going on. I studied his food diary. We talked about his family life.

Together we discovered it all came down to lunch.

Yes, lunch. It seems that Jack was one of four siblings, three boys and one girl. Whereas his brothers and sister were boisterous and energetic, he was quiet, studious. Their personalities carried through at dinnertime. While his siblings laughed and talked and shared stories of their day with their parents, Jack would sit, invisible, and eat. He'd eat and eat and eat, hoping no one would ask him a question. And at the same time hoping everyone would stop talking and ask him, really ask him, how he was and how he was doing.

These jumbled emotions made him blank out. He felt so bad that, yes, he ate his feelings rather than confront them.

As he grew up and became a highly visible defense lawyer, these eating patterns continued. He began to argue with the best of them, but at mealtime there was always the blank-out. Jack became a zombie.

Lunches with his colleagues. Dinner with his friends. Sunday-morning breakfast with his family. It didn't matter. Jack would shovel in the food, not noticing and not caring what it was he was eating.

This eating pattern earned him an extra one hundred pounds—and a *fathead* issue that would always be there to taunt him until we identified it, recognized it, and made a plan of action.

THE ADELE PUHN TWO-STEP PROGRAM:
IDENTIFY AND RECOGNIZE

I don't mean to make the *fathead* issues simplistic, as some of the above might imply. The *fathead* quiz as well as the "zombie" story are merely a way to get you thinking, to get you to identify and recognize your unique feelings so that you don't go off track. With a body that's in good blood sugar, you're more able to hear what your *fathead* is saying—and why.

And you'll be less afraid to deal with it—or to seek professional help if necessary. As one of my clients, a housewife and mother in her fifties, said, "This diet empowered me. Literally. Suddenly I was making decisions and choices based on what I wanted—not what my husband or children or friends wanted. I was able to understand my frustrations—and change them. A fifty-year-old in college? Why not!"

It's not difficult to see how the 5-Day Miracle Diet was connected to her finishing school. Not only did the facts that she felt tremendous energy, was able to concentrate more fully, and had newborn confidence in her slimmer frame help her reach her goals, but the very idea that she could succeed at something (the diet) made her feel she could succeed at something else: college. She became an active participant in life.

Think about it. Suddenly you're putting yourself first. You're saying, "I want to go to a different restaurant. I'll enjoy it more because of my diet." Or: "This fish is swimming in oil. Please take it back." You're making decisions, standing up for yourself. For many women this isn't just mind-boggling, it's completely empowering.

For my newly empowered client the *fathead* issues were very similar to those in other women I have helped. The need to please. Putting yourself last. Some of it had to do with habit. Some of it had to do with other people. And some of it had to do with her family life—and her fear that being thin and confident would force her to see how unhappy she'd been for years, stuck in a hausfrau role that didn't fulfill her needs—until of course she began to take a stand . . . for herself.

And sometimes the newfound confidence you have, once seemingly so threatening to a spouse, becomes a turn-on. How wonderful to be proud of the one you love!

Not every situation has such dramatic solutions. Not every client changes his or her life drastically when the *fathead* is identified and recognized. Sometimes people's subconscious fears are proven to be unfounded—and they go on with their work and their private lives just as before, but without that nagging, subtle doubt that was always present and made them eat. As with Jack, life goes on the way it always has—but with a bit more flair, a bit more joie de vivre, a bit more enthusiasm—and a lot less weight.

You may be staying in bad blood sugar so that you can be focused on your excess weight, using it as a distraction from your real disappointment with life. Unfortunately the bad blood sugar *contributes* to these feelings of pain. You're down, you're blue—and you need a distraction bad.

When you work at resolving these life issues, you'll be more likely to allow yourself to be in good blood sugar, and suddenly you're not as disappointed in yourself as you had been in your bad-blood-sugar state.

And with your newfound confidence brought on by GBS (good blood sugar), you need your distractions less and less. You're also ready to face your *fathead* head-on.

The Identification and Recognition Two-Step is a technique I have found extremely helpful in deleting saboteurs from the 5-Day Miracle Diet. The first step is to see what your *fathead* is up to. Examine your food diary; see the times of day and the situations where you found it particularly difficult to stay in GBS. Take a look around you, at what's going on at home, in the office, late at night. How do you feel when you overeat? Are you conscious of what you are doing? Is it nerves or is it habit? Or is it both?

Once you suspect what your *fathead* issues are, you can recognize what to do about it. When Jack realized he blanked out at mealtime (a behavior that had followed him throughout his life), he started wearing a rubber band around his wrist, under his shirt cuff. When he'd be ready to eat, he'd gently snap the rubber band—which not only startled him, but reminded him to watch what he ate. He made a conscious effort to listen to the other people around him. He would speak up and add to the conversation. And just as an extra consciousness-raising task, he also made sure he put his fork down on his plate in between bites; he *always* left at least one bite of food on his plate.

Perhaps your *fathead* sabotages you at snack time. Maybe you don't eat your hard chews at regular times. Once you identify the problem, you can recognize what to do—even if you don't yet know the deep-seated ramifications behind your actions. You can write a note to yourself and post it on your front door: "Don't forget snack!" You might use an alarm clock in your office. Perhaps you'll put all your hard chews on your desk as soon as you come in to work—and eat the first one before you begin your day.

Identify your *fathead* issues—and recognize them when they pop up. That's what the quiz—and this chapter—is all about. After all, the bottom line is that the *fathead* is still only 25 percent of your 5-Day Miracle Diet!

THE SIMPLE SABOTEURS

Identifying the simple saboteurs is not quite as simple as the name implies. By simple I mean close to the surface. These *fathead* issues are not buried too deeply.

Sublimating Anger, or "I Hate Him So Much That I'm Going to Eat This Entire Cake!"

One of my first clients was Martin. He was a well-dressed man in his forties, a successful salesman for a pharmaceutical firm with a wife and two children. He seemed eager to try the diet, but every week without fail he'd come in with a food diary that ensured he'd remain in bad blood sugar. Invariably I'd review his program with him and discuss what he was doing and why. I'd suggest ideas to help him in his competitive work environment. We discussed meditation, deep breathing, preparing food the night before, even finding a different job. Nothing. He'd come in and complain. He wanted to change the diet; he "sneaked" snacks. I kept trying to get him on the right track. I kept trying to explore with him what was wrong with the foods he was eating and he'd always counter with pride, almost bragging, "Yeah, but I could have been *really* bad. You should have seen the food I *didn't* eat."

This went on for two months. Finally I couldn't stand it anymore. I hated the idea that Martin was wasting his money coming to see me. It wasn't working. Something was keeping him from implementing the workable ideas and strategies we discussed in our sessions.

So I tried a different tack. I didn't go over the extra snacks or the wrong hard-chew timings. Instead I reassured him. I told him I was sure he was doing the best he could—and, after all, he could have done much worse.

Martin paused for a few moments. Finally he broke the silence. He asked me point-blank, "Are you angry with me?" I shook my head no. It almost seemed as if he *expected* me to be.

We started to talk—and I learned that his father always criticized him; he yelled at him and nagged him continuously, just as *his* father had done with him. He was angry at his father, but he couldn't admit it. Instead he "sneaked" around his anger—by sneaking food. He learned to "alibi." He couldn't hear what I was saying because he simply wasn't listening. He was alibiing, or rationalizing—just, it turned out, as he had done with his father to avoid confrontation. He took his anger out on food. When I asked him why he ate an extra snack or what he was feeling during our sessions when he forgot his hard chew, he saw my attempts at identification and recognition in the same light as those long-ago days with his father. He interpreted my help as criticism. What did he do? He focused his attention on an alibi, quickly making excuses to avoid examining the way he really felt. *He ate because he was angry at me.*

Once he identified and recognized this particular *fathead* issue, Martin was able to hear what I had to say. He no longer needed to alibi. He lost weight.

Recognizing your anger—and dealing directly with its source—will go a long way toward dissipating this *fathead*'s power.

Fear of Sexuality, or "I Look Too Sexy. I Must Be a Terrible Person."

Nancy loved her father. She was "Daddy's little girl" and she didn't care. Her father in turn doted on her. There was nothing he wouldn't do for Nancy; as far as he was concerned, there was nothing she couldn't do if she put her mind to it, and no one to compare with her. As Nancy approached puberty, she began to fill out. Her body took on a more womanly shape; she was losing her baby fat. Suddenly boys no longer seemed grotesque to her. There were even a few who were quite cute. And reading risqué novels with a flashlight at night became her—and her friends'—regular routine.

Nancy was growing up and, like any other normal teenager, she thought a lot about sex.

But there was a price to pay with this loss of innocence. When her father put his arm around her, she grew uncomfortable. She pulled away when he sat down next to her on the couch. Her father didn't understand Nancy's pulling back; there was no overt titillation going on. And Nancy, for her part, didn't understand why she felt uncomfortable. This was her father! She loved him!

Nancy began to eat—and eat. By the time she came to see me, she needed to lose sixty-five pounds. She was older—but not wiser. Once she was in good blood sugar, it took several months with her therapist for her to understand the unconscious oedipal anxieties that had been going on between her and her father, anxieties so abhorrent to face that she would rather eat and be fat than look sexy.

Recognizing her fear of sexuality turned her *fathead* into a thin—and sexy—head.

▲ ▲ ▲ ▲ ▲ ▲ ▲ ▲

FOOD / SEX

Safe sex is good. Feeling sexy can be exhilarating. Identifying and recognizing your fear of sexuality can be the best discovery in your life. It can turn your *fathead*—and your life—into a thin, sexy, and exciting one. Making love to a person you love is much more satisfying than making love to a hot fudge sundae. (You can even share one later, as an "Extra"!)

▼ ▼ ▼ ▼ ▼ ▼ ▼ ▼ ▼

Fear of Intimacy, or "I'll Show You. I'll Eat So Much That You'll Never Want to Get Close—and I'll Tell Myself It's All Your Fault. So . . . Pass the Bread Basket. Now!"

Lindsay was insecure and she'd been rejected by many men in the past. But it was difficult for me to see why when she came into my office. Lindsay, as the adage goes, had a beautiful face. She had a good sense of humor and an independent spirit. She earned her living as an editor and was very successful at her job. However, she was too heavy to be healthy. She needed to lose about twenty-five pounds.

"Of course no one wants to date me," she told me after her five days. "Look how fat I am!"

The fact was that Lindsay didn't *want* to date. She was afraid of intimacy. During our sessions she began to open up. It turned out that two years ago she'd been in love with a man who'd left her for her best friend. It hurt so much that she vowed she would never start dating again. She decided most definitely that it was *not* "better to have loved and lost than never to have loved at all." As far as she was concerned, if she never dated again, she'd be happy.

However, Lindsay wasn't happy. Not at all. Underneath her hurt, her pain, and her fear was a loving, giving person who desperately wanted to share her life with someone.

I reassured her and told her to keep going. Six months later Lindsay had lost twenty-five pounds. She was starting to look fabulous; men were beginning to notice her.

Bingo. At our next session she was suddenly in low blood sugar and two pounds heavier—even though she'd managed to be in good blood sugar for all those months!

We discussed Lindsay's motivation. She identified

her *fathead* issue: She was terrified of getting rejected again. It was like a sign emblazoned on a waving red flag: Better to be fat and distant. Now that she was beginning to date, all her old fears were cropping up—and coming out as a missed hard chew, a bad lunch, a binge at night. We recognized what she could do: Keep going. She talked to herself—and to her good friends—about her fears, and how the past was the past and it didn't have to repeat itself. She began to concentrate on feeling comfortable with her new look, the great clothes she'd recently bought, the ease with which she could get dressed, and a makeover she had scheduled at a department store. She was also scrupulous in writing in her food diary. By concentrating on the positive, nonthreatening results of her weight loss, she could overcome her internal fears.

Today Lindsay has reached her goal—and she's living with someone. Her *fathead* is buried in the past—where it belongs.

Distraction, or "If I Concentrate on These Five Pounds, I Won't Have to Concentrate on My Life."

Mary seemingly had it all. In fact when she opened the door to my office, I wondered why she was there. She was slim, well dressed, tall, and simply gorgeous. She smiled at me.

"This might sound silly, but I just can't seem to lose these last five pounds."

I agreed to work with her. If Mary wanted to lose five more pounds to help her image, I would help her reach her goal. I was there to help, not judge.

Within two weeks Mary was in good-blood-sugar heaven. She easily lost three pounds. Then something happened. Mary canceled her next appointment. She came in two weeks later and, sure enough, she had gained back the three pounds. She fussed and fretted and kept talking about her need to lose weight.

I looked at her and asked her directly, "Mary, this is not about weight. What don't you want to deal with?"

Mary sighed. She hesitated. And she began to talk. It turned out that she and her husband were having trouble. They seemed to be fighting all the time. They weren't connecting. They'd been married eighteen years and the very thought of separation gave her an anxiety attack. Obviously thinking about five pounds was a lot easier than thinking about her marriage.

For Mary her *fathead* issue lost its power when she faced it—"fat" head-on. She decided to feel her feelings instead of feeding them. She and her husband had a few sessions of marriage counseling. They decided to make appropriate changes and plans for a secure future . . . together.

Guilt, or "I'm a Terrible Person, I'll Take Some More, Please. . . . I Feel So Bad, Just a Little, No, a Little More, More."

Andy was one of my clients who came to me not to lose weight but to gain good health. He had ulcers and needed a special diet to keep his stomach calm. And as he said to me, "If I lost a few pounds, it wouldn't hurt."

Andy needed the diet. He was living through stressful times. His wife was off on the West Coast visiting their married daughter and he missed her. He was lonely. His son, of whom he'd been so proud, had just dropped out of college.

Andy soon had the tools to keep his condition—and in turn his stress—under control. He was in good blood sugar. But almost as soon as he got on the program, he got off. Week after week his food journal listed things he ate at night—after dinner.

Not only did these foods—fruits and angel food cake and ice milk—wreak havoc with his blood sugar, they also induced physical pain. They made his ulcer flare up.

It only took a few more sessions to recognize and identify Andy's *fathead* issues. He, too, used food as a distraction from the emotions raging inside. But he took it one step further: His loneliness stemming from his wife's absence and the guilt over the anger and disappointment he felt about his son's leaving school made him style his own brand of "hair shirt": an active ulcer.

Fear of Success, or "Sure, I Want the Corner Office. One Hamburger Platter to Go"

Susan had an MBA from a top school. She was determined to go to the top of a Fortune 500 company. She worked her way up, and five years later she was a vice president. It was at this juncture that she began to eat . . . and eat. With every accolade, every raise, she'd eat some more. Soon she was forty pounds overweight and feeling very much out of control.

After Susan got into good blood sugar and began to lose weight, she began to actually feel her feelings—instead of eating them. She realized that she was terrified of success, of the aggression she needed to get where she was.

But there was more. In addition to the "simple" fear there was deep-rooted motivation behind her behavior. Susan, like so many others, also had *fathead* issues that were much more complex.

Life Is Hard, or "I Deserve a Treat . . . and Another. . . ."

Being in a Recess State of Mind is a common saboteur. We stop making the effort for a meal, a day, a week, or a month. For many of us, vacations mean no-holds-barred. They mean forgetting your diet, forgetting good blood sugar, forgetting you ever heard the word *fathead*. I call this a Recess State of Mind because, as for a child in school, the recess bell means running out the doors screaming at the top of your lungs, "Free at last!" In fact my clientele dwindles during the summer months, only to come back at Labor Day like gangbusters—as if they were going back to school.

A Recess State of Mind also occurs between Thanksgiving and New Year's Day. As I tell my clients, this means that "Thanksgiving begins on the last Thursday of November and ends on New Year's Day." During these few months people are celebrating. They are having parties. They're not in school, and even if they are, they're certainly not doing any work! They're telling themselves, "After New Year's, I'll be able to . . ."

But it doesn't have to be this way. Wouldn't it be wonderful to appreciate your vacation or holidays with all your sensations intact? Wouldn't it be nice to enjoy the sun or the museum or the walk in the woods without the lethargy, depression, and sluggishness of bad blood sugar? Wouldn't it be fantastic to look sexy and vibrant during the holiday season?

I'm not saying you shouldn't enjoy yourself, I'm just asking you to go away or attend a celebration without a Recess State of Mind. Bring your string beans. Don't lose the basics of the program; even though you'll be eating more "Extras," you'll still wind up needing less and eating less.

THE PARTYHEAD

Are you a Partyhead, ready to play till you drop? If you are, you have a Recess State of Mind—but only when it comes to events: weddings, showers, bar mitzvahs, birthday parties. All mean carte blanche to eat what you want—and enough of it to make you happy.

Remember my Four Rules of Selectivity:

1. You must be in good blood sugar.
2. The food you choose must be appropriate.
3. The food must be something you really, really want.
4. You should eat as little of the "Food You Adore" as possible. You should eat just enough to satisfy your taste buds— whatever that amount may be.

It works—for daily living *and* for parties. Have that piece of cake! That glass of champagne! Those little hors d'oeuvres—whatever they are! If you follow my Rules of Selectivity, this particular brand of *fathead* won't stand a chance. You're armed and dangerous!

THE COMPLEX SABOTEURS

We live in the past. I don't mean that we live our lives dreaming of what was or what is no longer. Nor do I mean we live our lives to recapture the magic of our youth. No. Living in the past has to do with patterns, with actions that are repeated again and again, hoping this time, please, this time let it be right.

Let my mother love me.

Let my father approve of me.

Let me be the wonderful, perfect child my parents wanted me to be.

Let me do the right thing to get rid of the guilt and the anger I have toward my siblings.

Let me be a partner with my mother—not a competitor.

These are some of the emotions, the unfulfilled needs, that make up complex sabotage, the unconscious manipulation of food to re-create emotions from the past.

Like a deep, dark well, our needs grow dense with time. We forget what it was we needed as a child. We forget that we needed the hugs or the reassurance. Instead we remember how our father gave us that ubiquitous chocolate chip cookie when we cried. How our mother made a delicious meal when we made that football pass. How the messages got all mixed up between approval and disapproval: I bought you your favorite dessert. Don't eat too much. Like Donna and her mother, we play an unconscious game of need and loss, using food as the pawn that moves across the board.

FATHEAD DEPARTMENT: DOES THIS SOUND FAMILIAR?

When someone says the magic words "You've lost enough weight already," I believe them right off—and dig into the dessert a friend baked herself. I'll start eating whatever I want whenever I want. And I stop reading diet articles. After all, they don't pertain to me anymore!

THE DAUGHTER AND THE SIDESHOW MIRROR

Both Lily's mother and grandmother were slender, but Lily herself weighed over two hundred pounds. She didn't remember a time when she wasn't fat. "It was my role," she told me in my office as she maintained a state of good blood sugar, as the *fathead* kept trying to sabotage her hard-earned weight loss. "Joe, my brother, was the scholar; Marge, my sister, was the beauty; and I was the fat one." Lily kept her familial role, keeping it up even as she grew up, even as she became an adult and lived away from home. After all, being "the fat one" was the only role she knew. It was the only role she could play that provided security and comfort.

Her family was always on her case, telling her, cajoling her, screaming at her to lose weight. "It was my identity. I can barely remember my parents talking to me about anything else *but* my weight."

Lily continued to lose weight. Identifying and recognizing her *fathead* issues helped her get past them. She changed her hair, highlighting it with blond. She now wore red lipstick and clothes that showed off her figure— not hid it.

In fact one weekend, while visiting her mother, she wore a new silk blouse. Her mother admired it and wanted to try it on. "Mom," Lily said, "what are you talking about? It will be too big."

Just the opposite. When Lily's mother tried on the blouse, it was too small. So ingrained was Lily's identity in her family "fat" role that she still saw herself as heavy. She still saw her mother as being much slimmer than she was.

I made Lily stand in front of a full-length mirror. "Look. You are thin. You are thinner than your mother. Now, that doesn't mean you've lost your position in your family. It just means change. Your role is no longer the 'fatty.' You can still be supportive—*and* thin! It doesn't mean you can't be a good daughter or an integral part of your family."

With my help and several heart-to-heart conversations with her family, Lily finally understood. She no longer looked in the mirror and saw a distorted view.

THE BROKEN MIRROR

"Fat people living in thin bodies" is more than a cliché. A University of Pennsylvania study of men and women dieters found that the weight always came back on because they still saw themselves as fat.

LET THE PUNISHMENT FIT THE CRIME

Food is not always the weapon of choice. Sometimes it's the punishment for "imaginary" crimes, crimes that become a trigger to eat. Complex sabotages also include a dose of masochism. Listen to this progression:

1. My mother is constantly sending me mixed signals.
2. They make me feel angry and confused.
3. This anger makes me feel guilty.
4. I'm a horrible person.
5. I need to punish myself.
6. I'll get fat and kill two birds with one stone: feed my anger and make fat my crime and executioner.

Think about it. If you are fat, you can *really* hate yourself. You can *really* feel terrible about yourself and your life. It becomes a self-fulfilling prophecy.

FIGHTING BACK

Yes, food can be very powerful, but, like Donna, you can fight back. She couldn't change the way her mother thought, but she could change the way she reacted. Before she'd visit her mother, she'd mentally prepare herself, identifying and recognizing her *fathead* issues:

- Mother as competitor
- Guilt
- Anger
- Past family roles

She's still not at a point where she can laugh it off, but when her mother makes a remark about her weight, she can ignore it. "One day at a time. That's how I do it," she told me. "I try to stay in good blood sugar as much as possible. It's a powerful tool against the *fathead*. And each time I don't succumb, the stronger I become."

You, too, can fight your *fathead*. Begin by identifying and recognizing your particular brand of beast. You can do this in the following ways:

1. Get in good blood sugar so that you are chemically fit to handle your emotional and mental issues.
2. Examine your comments in your food journal.
3. Analyze your results from the *fathead* quiz.
4. Ask yourself what you are really feeling and feed yourself the appropriate *emotional* food.
5. Think back on recent situations. Ask yourself if you really wanted to eat that ice cream. Try to dig deep and discover what was really going on. Maybe you were having fun with your friends and you didn't want to be "singled out" as the dieter. Maybe you were angry that you were the only heavy one—and

that made you resentful enough to eat. Maybe you'd had a tough day at work and you were exhausted and sad.

6. Write your thoughts down in a notebook. Call it your personal *fathead*. No one has to know.

TECHNIQUES FOR IDENTIFYING AND RECOGNIZING FATHEAD ISSUES—AND GETTING RID OF THEM, TOO

The next time you find yourself reaching for a trigger-food "Extra," even though you are in good blood sugar, do the following:

1. Stop for a moment.
2. Ask yourself what you are really feeling.
3. Face the feeling—whatever it is.
4. Delay, delay, delay.

Delaying is a particularly good distraction for *fathead* beasts. When you are craving an inappropriate food, don't say no. Say wait . . . about twenty minutes. It's easier to say "Not yet" than "Not at all."

This delay breaks the pattern. It gives you a chance to discover what you are really feeling. It gives you time to analyze your feelings and to decide what you really want.

At this point you might realize that true fulfillment comes with emotional food, such as a call to a friend, rather than with rocky road ice cream. You will feed your emotional hunger with the appropriate food.

Sometimes this twenty-minute delay is all you need to dissipate the craving and help you recognize what you really want. However, if you still feel the urge, make a "deal" with yourself. Have a carrot or any other hard chew. If that still doesn't work, go for a "Quick Fix."

Then, if all else fails, have as little as possible of the food you're craving to feel satisfied.

And, most important, relax. Go on with your life! Everything is a learning experience, including identifying and recognizing your *fathead*. This, too, will lose its power over you.

Once you've done the *fathead* two-step—identifying and recognizing—you'll be able to "own" the 5-Day Miracle Diet. No one will be able to take it away. It's yours: a healthy, energetic, optimistic way of life. Let's go on to the strategies that make ownership a reality.

CHAPTER 6

"Owning" the 5-Day Miracle Diet

When I set 160 as my weight goal, I would have settled for the high 160s. I really never expected to see 160 (never mind pass it on my way down)!
—A twenty-seven-year-old teacher

I can write the letter now:

Dear Adele,
I feel great! I spent five days getting my blood sugar under control and I've been in good blood sugar for weeks now. I've examined my fathead issues and there's no doubt about it, I'm a "Sugarbaby" through and through. I'm probing deeper, though, and discovering more and more about myself—and about other people's sabotage.

But I'm getting nervous. What next? How do I make this diet my own? How can I be sure I take it with me wherever I go? How do I make it stick?
In Good Blood Sugar but Nervous

Dear Nervous,
Read this chapter and you'll do fine!

PERSPECTIVE TIME

I don't allow the words *good* and *bad* when clients describe themselves based on how they've eaten the past week. Eating does not make you a good or a bad person. As I've asked my clients when they tell me they've been "bad," "Did you just commit a hit-and-run? Did you just rob an elderly lady?" Now, that's bad. And it doesn't have a thing to do with food.

OWNING THE DIET AT WORK

Benjamin is a vice president of a Fortune 500 company. He's extremely goal oriented; he's a brilliant problem solver. Bring him any question about budget, presentation, employee relations, or marketing and he'll answer it. But, as straight thinking as Benjamin was, when it came to his 5-Day Miracle Diet plan, he kept hitting a blood-sugar wall. If he was in a meeting, he wouldn't eat his hard chew; he couldn't keep his mealtime hours. Here's how I told him to own the diet at work:

- Bring carrots or any other hard chews into your meetings to ensure that you have your two-hour chew.
- Discreetly keep your hard chews in your desk drawer. Eat your carrot *before* the meeting begins.
- Pack your snacks in plastic bags for work the night before. Even if you have to run out the door, you'll have time to grab them from the fridge. Put a note on the front door so that you don't forget them!
- Excuse yourself from the meeting. Instead of going to the rest room, go to your office and eat your chews.
- Grab a quick, but appropriate, breakfast before you

leave the house: a slice of bread and a slice of cheese, a rice cake spread with a little peanut butter, a slice of chicken and a slice of bread.

- If you're not accustomed to eating breakfast, decide what you're going to have the night before. Like thinking about what you're going to wear, it will make the process fast and easy.

- Bring your hard and soft chews with you in your attaché case, next to your appointment book and files (in plastic wrap, of course!).

- Eat your snacks on the run, in a taxi, in between meetings, driving your car—in short, as often as you need to eat them—as long as you also eat your controlled soft- or hard-chew snacks at the right time.

- *You* make the lunch plans—and pick a restaurant where you can maintain your good blood sugar: Japanese, continental, seafood, almost anyplace will do if you want to stay on track!

- Eat small amounts of hard-chew vegetables before you walk into the restaurant for lunch in case none are available. This way you'll keep your blood sugar stabilized and you won't be tempted.

- Set a timer so that you won't be so caught up with work that you'll forget your hard chews.

- Plan ahead: Shop for food for the week on the weekend, or one weekday night. Do quick fill-ins at the greengrocer on your way home for stocking up on fresh produce.

- Think convenient: washed baby carrots, precut and cleaned cauliflower and broccoli, salad mixes, Chinese takeout that consists of tofu and steamed veggies.

- Spend your free lunch hours at the gym—or get a manicure or facial. Treat yourself well. You deserve it!

OWNING THE DIET AT PARTIES

Ellie's best friend asked her to be a bridesmaid at her
wedding in two months' time. Ellie was pleased with the
honor, but she was also terrified. How could she fit into
one of those feminine gowns; she couldn't lose the
twenty pounds in time for the first fitting! And how could
she go to the wedding? There would be a cocktail hour,
appetizers, wedding cake. Impossible! She became more
and more distraught as the big day arrived. Here are
some of the suggestions I gave Ellie so that she could
own the 5-Day Miracle Diet plan at the wedding—and at
any party:

- Let everyone else go to the buffet table first. By the
  time you get there, it won't look as appetizing.
- Look over *all* the hors d'oeuvres before choosing any for
  yourself. If many of them look fabulous, make them your
  dinner—or have a few as "Extras." Use your protein and
  starchy carbohydrate allotment. When you do sit down to
  dinner, simply fill up on salad and vegetables. (And, yes,
  you can take a *small* bite of a protein and starch if the dinner looks great, too! It won't hurt you and you'll enjoy
  the party so much more.)
- Just say no when the waiter comes around carrying a
  tray. He or she will be long gone before you've even
  smelled what was on the platter.
- Make yourself a Virgin Mary extra hot. The spiciness
  will make you feel a buzz.
- Nurse a white-wine spritzer—after you've had a plain
  seltzer. This way you'll be able to walk into the room
  without immediately responding to the environmental
  cue "Oh, a party. Give me a drink." The plain seltzer in
  your hand will keep the champagne server away; it will
  keep you in control so that you decide whether or not

you'll have alcohol for the next round. (And after all, you have only two hands!)

- Avoid sugary mixed drinks. Piña coladas, margaritas, whiskey sours—these are all double whammies: full of refined sugar *and* alcohol.
- Hang out as far away from the food and bar as possible.
- If you hear the music, dance!
- Eat a hard chew before walking in the door, either in your car or in a taxi or a bus. It will make you feel full and balanced.
- Eat a light dinner with lots of vegetables, including only half of your protein (the allotted amount). This way you can eat two or three more ounces of protein, starch, and some more vegetables at the party without getting off track.
- Make the party one of your "Foods You Adore" situations. Decide what you really, really want to eat or drink and enjoy!
- Decide beforehand which two categories of "Foods You Adore" you'll want to stick with. This way the array of food and drink won't be too overwhelming. You'll zero right in on the caviar and the stuffed mushrooms—and/or the fabulous desserts.
- Wear something that shows off your new shape. (And if all the compliments make you feel threatened rather than fantastic, think of it this way: You've just discovered another *fathead* issue to work on!)
- Go to the party in good blood sugar. Eat properly for two days *before* the event. You'll not only be the life of the party, full of vitality and joie de vivre, but you'll be amazed at how little the party fare will tempt you.
- Alcohol is not a particularly good choice. It's a real trigger, and after one or two drinks, you won't care about good blood sugar (until the next morning, of course!).

- If you bite into a "Food You Adore" that looks absolutely scrumptious but turns out to be absolutely horrible, get rid of it! Period.
- If you go to a party and your blood sugar is only so-so, immediately head for the crudités and start chomping (sans dip, of course!).

GOOD PARTY FARE / BAD PARTY FARE

GOOD CHOICES

- Caviar
- Crudités
- Smoked salmon
- Sashimi, or, if you need the rice, some sushi—but not as much!
- If you must have a drink, a better choice is a wine spritzer
- Mineral water
- Stuffed grape leaves
- Salsa with plain bread or crackers
- Steamed dumplings
- Skewered beef or chicken

NOT-SO-GOOD CHOICES (BUT STILL ALLOWED)

- Pigs-in-blankets
- Cheese, especially the high-fat delights such as Brie and Saint André
- Cream cheese or sour cream
- Tiny egg rolls
- Fried dumplings
- Hard liquor
- More than one or two glasses of wine—you'll lose your resolve!

OWNING THE DIET WHEN YOU ARE IN A RESTAURANT

Lately whenever anybody asked Jared to join them for lunch or dinner out, he always had an excuse. He was getting the reputation of being a tightwad and a spoilsport. Unfortunately the only person who was spoiling his fun was Jared himself. He'd been on the 5-Day Miracle Diet for three months; he was losing weight at a steady clip, one to two pounds a week. But to Jared the word *diet* was synonymous with *suffer*. He had to sacrifice. He had to eat plain, tasteless foods. Even when it was time for a "Food You Adore," he'd stick to an exotic salad or an extra fruit. I told Jared that he didn't have to go to an Italian restaurant and order dry fish. He could eat out and enjoy it. Here are some other suggestions I gave him:

- Immediately ask for a green salad sans dressing or some crudités.
- Ask that the rolls be taken away—or at least place them near someone who isn't dieting.
- If you feel tempted, simply taste your colleague's fattening entrée. If you're in good blood sugar, it will be enough.
- Use the occasion for a "Food (or Drink) You Adore."
- Order first—that way you won't be tempted when you hear what others are getting.
- Choose fresh fruit for dessert.
- Ask for your salad dressing on the side.
- Eat a hard chew before going to the restaurant.
- Even though everyone thinks Japanese food is lo-cal, it can be hazardous to your GBS health. Miso soup contains a lot of salt. Sushi packs a lot of rice. A better choice is sashimi with rice on the side. Or ask for sushi made with less rice.
- Try to plan dinner at a reasonable hour so that you'll

maintain your good blood sugar. If dinner's at eight, make sure you have your hard chew.

- Try to eat in restaurants where dining out isn't a challenge. (Even the finest French restaurants have delicious grilled chops and vegetables.) If the waiter gets your entrée wrong, send it back without making a scene. If necessary, order some soup and a plain baked potato so that your friends or colleagues aren't waiting for you. It makes awkwardness a thing of the past.

THE MAN WHO LOVED CHAMPAGNE

One of my clients, a gentleman of about fifty, had been in good blood sugar for weeks. When I asked him what challenges he had coming up, he shrugged his shoulders. "Oh, well, I guess, there's the wedding. But I don't consider that a challenge."

I looked at him. "Wedding? You don't consider that a challenge?"

"No."

We reviewed his journal the day after the wedding. Sure enough, he had had crudités and a plain entrée. He didn't even have a bite of cake.

I smiled. I was delighted for him. But I was worried, too. Was he being too strict with himself? Would the *fathead* rear up because it was feeling deprived?

My client shook his head. He was in good blood sugar and had no cravings. He chose not to eat at the wedding. Why? That week he was spending his birthday with a friend he hadn't seen in years. He planned a night of "Food You Adore." He chose vodka and caviar (without the sour cream). He intended on eating his favorite hors d'oeuvres and drinking his favorite schnapps in his favorite restaurant—and making merry all night. The wedding the week before wasn't the least bit tempting.

Planning—in good blood sugar—makes perfect!

OWNING THE DIET WHEN TRAVELING
ON BUSINESS OR PLEASURE

Joan couldn't wait for her vacation. She had been on the 5-Day Miracle Diet for only three weeks, but she already looked and felt fabulous. Although she was in great blood sugar, I was worried. She seemed to be losing weight solely for her trip, a cruise to the Caribbean. She wasn't thinking past the white bikini she bought. I was afraid that she'd get on the boat, bring her luggage to her cabin, then let the fun begin! I was certain she'd be in a Recess State of Mind, deciding that dieting was "work" and, like summer vacation in school, she was at play. Here are some of the suggestions I gave her, tips and hints that could be used for both pleasurable vacations and business travel:

- Pack your baby carrots and other hard chews in plastic bags along with your socks and shoes.
- Scout out the health food stores in your area. Tofu and rice cakes make a great breakfast!
- By all means order room service—but be selective. Don't just ask for crudités. Ask for crudités consisting of two carrots, six radishes, and four broccoli florettes.
- Take advantage of the hotel's gym and pool. Always pack exercise gear, athletic shoes, and shorts. In today's world of stretchy synthetics, they don't take up much room.
- If you're traveling for fun, remember to avoid the Recess State of Mind. Pack your carrots and do the best you can!
- Think about having one "Extra" every day while you're away, preferably at dinner, when you've spent a whole day in good blood sugar. You'll be less likely to splurge extravagantly.

- If you eat the right breakfast, snacks, and lunch, you're ahead of the game. I guarantee you won't binge at dinner—even if you eat a "Food You Adore" every night you're away.
- Think *maintaining* your weight, not losing or gaining.
- Think of good blood sugar as money in the bank. It's there; it's keeping you secure; you can withdraw from it whenever you want. This means you should absolutely have the pasta in Italy, the wine in Portugal, the steak in Chicago. By staying in or getting back into good blood sugar again, you make a "deposit" and your "savings account" stays even—or goes up.

A TRAVELIN' WOMAN

One of my clients was going on her first trip to Paris. She was ecstatic and couldn't wait to get there. Of course she was ready to eat à la française—but she did bring her carrots on the plane. She and her husband went with another couple who were not on the 5-Day Miracle Diet. They didn't bring any carrots. In fact they laughed at my client. While they ate their croissants and coffee for breakfast, my client searched out apples. She ate a delicious piece of nine-grain bread. Consequently by four o'clock in the afternoon the other couple was in dire need of a nap—after eating some French chocolates. But my client was still rarin' to go. She and her husband took a long, lingering walk on the Seine. And that evening? The other couple fell asleep right after their heavy dinner. But my client and her husband went to the Champs Élysées and danced the night away!

Now, who do you think had the better time?

OWNING THE DIET WHEN EATING AT
A FRIEND OR RELATIVE'S HOUSE

Lenore always had trouble saying no—especially when it came to food. Whenever she dined at a friend's house, she always asked for seconds; she loved the pleasure she saw in her host's eyes. And at family gatherings? Lenore was footloose and fancy-free, like always. Her large family always enjoyed sitting around the dining room table, eating and drinking and laughing half through the night. When she'd been on my program for two weeks, we began talking about "other people's food" and what it meant to her. I helped her see that she could be a welcome guest without eating seconds—and she could enjoy the love of her family without an extra helping of cake. Here are some of the suggestions I gave her:

- When your friend says she or he "slaved" for hours over dessert, say no with love and passion in your voice. "It looks fabulous. I am having such an incredibly good time sitting here and enjoying your meal and the wonderful conversation. You're such a wonderful cook! I feel so perfect that I just want to sit here for a while. I just want to wait before I eat another thing." By the time everyone's eaten, they will have forgotten that you didn't have a piece of that soufflé.
- Choose this night for a "Food You Adore" situation.
- When your host asks you if you want seconds, always remember to compliment him or her before saying how full you are.
- Relatives can be particularly sensitive. When your aunt Ida tells you she made your favorite dessert, lemon meringue pie, give her a hug. Tell her she's great and that you'll take a piece later. (The hug and the appreciation, after all, is what she was looking for in the first place.)

- If it's a close friend or relative, call up in advance and find out what's for dinner or offer to bring a veggie side dish. It can help you plan.
- Keep your diet to yourself. Beware well-meaning but hidden saboteurs!
- Remember, you can't change people, but you can change the way you cope with situations. You don't have to explain *why* you're not having seconds on the baked Alaska.

OWNING THE DIET FOR PERSONAL GROWTH

Mark couldn't believe it when I told him that eating poorly would be the exception, not the rule, when he was on the 5-Day Miracle Diet. An architect who often stayed up all night, lost in his ideas for buildings, he frequently ate quick snacks—junk food that could be unwrapped and eaten fast. But I promised him that he would lose the desire to eat junk food, that he would opt for a Twinkie less and less. And even if he did gobble the occasional cupcake, he would recover much faster. He'd become more adept at returning to a good-blood-sugar state. He'd have the tools and the knowledge, and most important the desire, to be in that wonderful, fabulous state called good blood sugar. Three months later Mark was eating red cabbage and cauliflower late at night; he kept them in plastic bags near his blueprints. Here are some of the suggestions for personal growth that I gave him during this time:

- Analyze a situation before plunging in: "Am I really hungry? Or am I feeling pressured? What am I *really* feeling? Do I really want to eat that cheesecake?"
- Distract yourself. If that cheesecake is calling out to you, reach out—for a supportive friend. If, after a

phone call, you still want your cake, well, you can eat
it, too—but just enough to satisfy yourself!

- Learn to take control over yourself. After all, you can't
control others, why not yourself? This is particularly
difficult for women who've been raised to please. But
taking charge is empowering. Try it. You'll like it.
Start with a restaurant. If the waiter got your order
wrong, send it back!

- Individualize the program—and don't be boring! For
example:

  If you like movie popcorn, make sure you treat yourself to a feature movie once a week and eat that
  "Food You Adore."

  If you find you can't live without a banana, try limiting
  it to only half—once in a while. And never use that
  half a banana for a control chew snack, and never eat
  it in the morning.

  If you need your caffeine, drink your coffee, but try to
  go half and half: half decaf, half regular. Wean yourself off of caffeine; it's mostly habit. Try an unfla-
  vored decaf coffee or unsweetened herbal tea in the
  afternoon.

- Revamp your negative thinking. Here's a spin your
brain can take:

Being in good blood sugar is a choice I've made.
I feel wonderful in good blood sugar.
I have so much energy!
Since I've lost weight, I go out much more.
I'm not ashamed to be seen—by anyone.
I'm loaded with confidence.
Is losing all this worth that chocolate chip cookie? No way!

OWNING THE DIET WHEN YOU'RE UNDER STRESS

Rita had an impossible deadline. A fashion editor of a top magazine, she was told she had to come up with a new cover and feature in two weeks. She tried to think—and drew a blank. She brainstormed with her staff, but couldn't come up with anything better than yet another Cindy or Kate cover. She couldn't sleep; she couldn't concentrate. And forget about her hard-chew snacks! She was so nervous that every *fathead* issue that ever entered her mind and soul came into play. Instead of carrots, she had cookies. She ate all night long. Now she had two problems: the cover and her weight gain. Rita had been on my program for over six months at this point. From our weekly sessions she knew what she had to do (in addition to coming up with a fabulous idea!) to overcome her overeating while under stress. Here's what she did—and what you can do, too:

- As with people, you can't change a stressful situation, but you can change the way you handle it!
- Say to yourself, "I can't ease the pain with food— at least not in the long run." If you eat under stress, you'll have two problems: the situation that caused the stress to begin with *and* the stress you feel by going off track . . . and being in bad blood sugar.
- If you're at work or you have only minutes to spare, try this quick relaxer: Sit up straight in your chair. Turn off the phone. Close your eyes. Take a deep breath. Another one. That's good. Another one. Take five deep breaths in all, counting deeply to ten on inhaling and ten on exhaling. Open your eyes. That's it! I bet you feel better already!
- Try other nonfood relaxation techniques. Some examples:

Meditation

Creative visualization tapes

Massage

Curling up with a good book or movie

Taking the dog out for a walk

Taking a bath with lots of stress-reducing oil

Talking to a supportive friend

Exercise! Take a walk. Go to the gym. Ride a bike. Try a yoga class.

Put on some relaxing music and close your eyes.

Go to a museum or sit in a park in the sunlight.

LESS IS NOT MORE

One more thing: *Never* eat less than the basic 5-Day Miracle Diet. You want to be healthy, strong, and in great blood sugar always!

THERE IS NO SUCH THING AS A RELAPSE: AN IMPORTANT PART OF OWNING THE 5-DAY MIRACLE DIET

If you own a house (or pay your mortgage on time), no one can take it away from you. If you own a car, it's yours. Similarly if you own this diet plan, it's yours—forever. It can't be taken away from you. Therefore it doesn't matter if you relapse. The cookie you just ate is part of your program—as an "Extra." Ditto the chef's salad at lunch or the pommes frites at dinner. So what if you overate? No one's keeping score. Instead of feeling hopeless and helpless, just accept what you've done; it's okay. You can do something about it because you are in control. Think of the times you eat more than the "Foods You Adore" as a learning experience. It will build your confidence as you get back on track. Remember, you can feel the effects of bad blood sugar anywhere from immediately to forty-eight to seventy-two hours *after* you've eaten, so you might not feel the results of that fattening dessert for two whole days!

The best solution? Get right back on track. Get out your food journal and write down what you ate. Exercise more the next day. Get back to basics—and be strict with your hard and soft chews. Try some stress-reducing exercises. Above all, don't beat yourself up!

After all, it would be like beating up on your house or your car or even your dog. You *own* my diet and it can't be taken away. Period.

WARNING: YOU ARE ABOUT
TO ENTER A *FATHEAD* STATE

- I've been thinking about the muffins downstairs in the coffee shop all morning.
- I'm not seeing my family until Friday night, and I'm already tense!
- I'm going on a cruise in two weeks. I'll never be able to stick to the plan.
- I am working too, too hard.
- It seems like I've been taking care of my entire family forever—and no one has done anything for me!
- I feel needy.
- I just broke up with my significant other.
- I'm really PMSing.
- My child just told me he/she doesn't want to go to college.
- I'm angry—but I don't know at what!

If any of these statements ring true, be aware that you're feeling vulnerable. Make sure you write in your food journal. Try to stick to the basics. Avoid tempting situations and difficult people. The feeling will pass. Delaying a so-called relapse is always better than starting one. It breaks the mood and builds confidence. Feed the need with a non-food strategy.

❦ ❦ ❦ ❦ ❦ ❦ ❦ ❦ ❦

Before we go on to the next chapter, I have one more thing to say to all you "food sensualists" out there. Like me, you enjoy food. It's wonderful. It's an important part of life. When my clients eat a "Food They Adore," I ask them to describe it, to tell me where they ate it, what it felt like, how much they enjoyed it.

I say the same to you. Enjoy yourself.

Just don't forget your carrots.

● ● ● ● ● ● ● ● ●

THE 5-DAY MIRACLE DIET
MAINTENANCE PLAN

People view maintenance as a magical place, a fairyland where their goals have all been met. My clients will ask me, almost awestruck, "What is maintenance like?"

The answer is easy. Maintenance is exactly what you are doing now. The 5-Day Miracle Diet is all about "practicing maintenance." It's a lifestyle, a program that goes with you wherever, forever, whenever. Once you own the plan, it's yours.

All you have to do when you've reached a place where you feel content with your weight is to simply increase the amount of food you are eating so that you can maintain your weight.

Continue to "eat thin." In other words, don't give up the mechanics of your diet plan. "Maintenance" does not mean "mindless." Don't go back to your old habits. Try not to eat at night after dinner. Keep consumption of "Food You Adore" to twice a week.

You must still eat your hard- and soft-chew snacks and your meals should still be eaten on the same schedule. But you can eat more. If you are not a carbohydrate addict, starches are a nice place to begin to increase your food intake. Add a starchy carbohydrate once a day every day or, if you'd rather, add another fruit instead. Or, if you're a protein person, increase your protein two or three ounces every day. Above all, do not forget the good blood sugar (GBS) that got you here to begin with.

WOMEN

Week One

- Add one additional starchy carbohydrate every day.
- Three times a week, on alternating days (say, Monday, Wednesday, and Friday) you can have a sandwich at lunch instead of a starchy carbohydrate at dinner.
- Or, on those same alternating days, add a third fruit instead of a carbohydrate.
- On the days you do not eat a sandwich, you can have, say, ⅔ cup rice (instead of ½ cup) or a slightly larger bowl of bean soup.
- If insulin-resistant, eat 2 ounces extra protein instead of the starch every day.
- You can also add a little more olive oil to your food or extra salad dressing.

Week Two

- If you have not gained any weight, or are still losing, you should continue this same regimen; however, in addition . . .
- Once or twice a week add one of the following: a small handful of raw almonds, 1 cup plain popcorn, or a handful of unsalted pretzels.

- If you find you are starting to gain weight, reduce these "Extras" to once a week, or once every two weeks.

Week Three and Onward

- Continue this regimen, "shooting the scale" once a week.
- If still losing, add another starchy carbohydrate or one fruit.
- If insulin-resistant, add a protein, another fruit, or a moderate portion of starchy carbohydrate (½ cup) on a nightly basis only.
- If gaining weight, cut back on the week-two "Extras."
- If still gaining, remove the extra protein.
- If still gaining, remove the starchy carbohydrate or the fruit.
- Don't forget to exercise to keep those metabolic fires burning!

MEN

Week One

- Add one additional starchy carbohydrate every other day.
- On alternating days (say, Monday, Wednesday, and Friday) you may add one fruit.
- You can have two breads at lunch in the form of a sandwich or 1½ cups starchy carbohydrate portion at lunch or dinner.
- If insulin-resistant, add 2 extra ounces protein instead of the starch every other day.
- You can also add a little more olive oil to your food or extra salad dressing.

Week Two

- If you have not gained any weight, or are still losing, you should continue this same regimen; however, in addition . . .
- Once or twice a week add one of the following "Extras": a small handful of raw almonds, 1 cup plain popcorn, or a handful of unsalted pretzels.

- If you find you are starting to gain weight, reduce these "Extras" to once a week, or once every two weeks.

Week Three and Onward
- Continue this regimen, "shooting the scale" once a week.
- If still losing, add another starchy carbohydrate or one fruit.
- If insulin-resistant, add protein or another fruit instead.
- If gaining weight, cut back on the week-two "Extras."
- If still gaining, remove the extra protein.
- If still gaining, remove the starchy carbohydrate or the fruit.
- Don't forget to exercise to keep those metabolic fires burning!

These numbers are not etched in stone. If you begin to exercise more, you might find that you are still losing weight. In such cases I suggest adding another week-two "Extra" until your weight has stabilized.

Remember, you own this program; it is your life. Experiment. Live! Try adding healthful, low-fat foods that you might not ever have tried before. Eat your extra fruit with enjoyment. Try different grains or a pita-pocket sandwich at lunch. Dip your "Extra" pretzels in mustard. Try salsa on your baked potato. In other words, don't think too much about it. Just live, and because you are in good blood sugar, your diet will take care of itself.

DIETING THROUGH HISTORY

Victorian women didn't need to say no to those hefty platters of meat and fowl. They simply spent two hours before dinner "lacing up," that is, donning a corset whose whalebones pushed in the skin and muscles (and bodily organs) and actually made waists up to six inches smaller! Of course these same women unfortunately had livers, stomachs, and lungs pushed out of proportion, and many women died of "corset disease."

CHAPTER 7

If You Are Insulin Resistant or a Carbohydrate Addict, Read This Now!

Adele, you changed my life. Period.
—A forty-year-old sales manager and
father of three

"What!!!!"

My client, a successful cinematographer, seemed to be in front of the camera—instead of behind its lens.

"No way!"

He picked up his attaché case, grabbed his coat, and was halfway out my office door.

"Gregory," I said calmly, sitting in my chair, my hands in my lap. "We're not talking life or death here."

We were talking pasta, or rather the need to eat less of it, which, I suppose, can be a matter of life or death for some.

It was for Gregory. (And, I have to confess, it was for me at one time, too.)

"Pasta, Gregory," I said. "And it's not all the time."

Gregory sighed. Suddenly he became the responsible thirty-six-year-old he really was. He sat his sturdy six-foot frame back in the chair, tossing his jacket on the floor.

"You're right, you're right." He ran his fingers through his hair. "For a minute I was back at the beginning, back to low-blood-sugar days."

I smiled. I knew how Gregory felt. He had been on the

5-Day Miracle Diet for six weeks now. The first three weeks he did great, losing weight, feeling incredible energy, losing his food urges. He'd kept a food diary, and even though he was currently shooting a film, he brought his carrots and apples to location.

Unfortunately by the fourth week Gregory had stopped losing weight. He'd lost a total of eleven pounds when we did "shooting the scale," but for the last two weeks he hadn't lost anything. And he still wanted to lose an additional fifteen pounds; he still had what he called a "diet Pepsi belly."

I knew the signs. I was one myself. Gregory was a carbohydrate addict.

And I had just told him that he couldn't eat pasta more than twice a week.

▲   ▲   ▲   ▲   ▲   ▲   ▲   ▲   ▲

THE SUGARBABY

I affectionately call these clients my Sugarbabys. They are all intelligent, successful, sophisticated adults, but they will still act like a six-year-old child when they think "mommy" isn't watching. This means candy, chocolate, Gummi Bears, peppermint, cotton candy, you name it. If it has sugar, they'll eat it.

This baby *loves* sugar. And it's especially prevalent in carbohydrate addicts. (Yes, all those simple carbohydrates and refined sugars dancing in your head.) If you're a Sugarbaby, you'll crave sugar all the time. When it comes to the "Food You Adore" once or twice a week, you'll go for the dessert every time. Even when you're in good blood sugar, the Sugarbaby remains a tempting red flag. Just looking at a pound cake puts on a pound. Chocolate talks to you. Sugarplums dance around in your head.

Not to worry. Identifying and recognizing this as a chemical issue prepares you. You can make a choice: the dessert at the restaurant Friday night instead of the Sara Lee on the way home from a bad day at work.

❦　❦　❦　❦　❦　❦　❦　❦　❦

INSULIN RESISTANT: A REALITY FOR SOME

On Wednesday, February 8, 1995, *The New York Times* had the story on the front page: SO IT MAY BE TRUE AFTER ALL: EATING PASTA MAKES YOU FAT. Suddenly, after a decade of a food pyramid consisting primarily of carbohydrates, it seemed all wrong. We were back to the days of Stillman and Atkins and high protein, no bread.

The article took the country by storm. Soon papers from coast to coast reported on the "dangers" of carbohydrates. Even prime-time news shows got into the act.

This led to a spate of books about carbohydrate addiction, and carbohydrates (even tricolored pasta, whole-grain bread, whole-wheat rolls, and other yummy, seemingly healthy complex carbs) became the new "no-no" in diet circles.

People began turning their noses away from carbohydrates, that once-safe haven and largest portion of the food pyramid. Pasta shelves in supermarkets were fated to get dusty. Breads—even those crunchy, nutty, seven-grain varieties—would go moldy in their plastic wrappers. You no longer had to wait for a table at your favorite Italian restaurant. Yes, bread and pasta were ready to become a thing of the past, up there with butter, eggs, sugar, Scotch whiskey, steak, and nicotine.

Sorry, wrong number.

THE TRUTH BEHIND THE
"BAN CARBOHYDRATES NOW!" PARADE

Yes, it's true that certain people are insulin resistant, or "carbohydrate addicts." What this means in real terms is that insulin, the hormone produced by the body to process sugar and starches, does not act normally when carbohydrates are eaten. Cells become resistant; they won't take the food inside. The body sends out more insulin, still trying to process those carbs. The result? Insulin is *overproduced*. This overabundance of insulin has nowhere to go; the cells in the body have been satiated. A message is sent to the brain: "Yoo-hoo, we need more carbs." We have all this excess insulin and it's telling us, "More, send in more carbs. More. More (e.g., the whole box of cookies). We crave. We want. We're addicted."

Unfortunately the carbohydrates the body now craves and *must* ingest stimulate *even more* insulin production. This excess insulin creates havoc in the body, increasing the appetite and the storage of fat.

Worse, the person has no choices. He or she is an addict. Like a smoker who is told to quit, the carbohydrate addict goes into a panic. As Gregory said, "Not my pasta!"

Unfortunately dieting alone doesn't cut it. A person who is insulin resistant or carbohydrate addicted can try to lose weight with the standard low-fat, high-carbohydrate diet plan and fail. In fact he or she can eat standard low-calorie, high-carbohydrate meals for the rest of his or her life—and still gain weight.

There is some good news: This chemical phenomenon occurs in only 25 percent of the people who are overweight. However, if you're one of them, the statistic hardly matters.

TO BE OR NOT TO BE INSULIN RESISTANT

Gregory is one of those 25 percent. So am I. This only means one-quarter of the overweight American population, but if you happen to be in that select group, it's difficult to give those carbohydrates up.

If you *are* a carbo-addict and in bad blood sugar, within forty-eight hours of carbo deprivation the cravings for pasta will become so intense that you will either remain white-knuckled and miserable for another two days or you'll immediately break down and eat an excess amount of thin spaghetti no. 9.

The biochemical conductor orchestrating this uncontrollable behavior feels like the selfsame bad-blood-sugar monster that was in place before you began the 5-Day Miracle Diet.

So . . . what do you do?

TO THINE OWN SELF BE TRUE

I suspected Gregory was a carbohydrate addict from the beginning because of his passion for pasta and bagels, but I had to be sure. The only way to know for sure without having a medical blood workup done is to wait.

Yes, wait.

Your body has to get into good blood sugar before you can know anything about carbohydrates. Before those five days of balancing your body you're like a craving machine: cookies, pasta, anything will do so long as it's *food*. But once your blood sugar is stabilized, you can begin to see what you *really* like and what you *really* don't. You'll no longer be dictated to by your bad blood sugar. You can see, clearly and easily, whether you are a pasta diva or not.

JOB ALERT!

According to an article in the *Los Angeles Times*, if you're a woman over forty, avoid carbs before a job interview. They'll make you sleepy and forgetful. On the other hand, if you're a man over forty, that same bowl of pasta will make you calm.

And if you happen to be a carbohydrate addict, you'll go past calm into unconsciousness, especially if you have pasta at lunch!

CARBO CRAVINGS, GO AWAY

Believe it or not, there is life after pasta. In fact, if you follow my special program for carbohydrate addiction, your cravings will simply go away. Suddenly you won't care if you eat that pasta or that roll or that bagel. You will no longer behave like an addict.

Of course right now the addict in you is saying, "No way! I'm not going to do it." But wait. If you're in good blood sugar and you strip the carbs from your meals, except bread for breakfast, for five days, you will soon see a tremendous difference. By the third or fourth day you're starting to feel great. You're

- Detached from food. You feel freer than you ever have in your life!
- No longer bloated. Your digestive system is clearer; you no longer have that "Pillsbury Doughboy look."
- Thinking much more clearly. In fact you're in a *fabulous* mental and physical state.
- Losing weight easily. Your face, your stomach, your buttocks and thighs—all of you *looks* thinner and more toned!

• Your stomach feels flatter and you have fewer digestive disturbances.

I can tell you all these things, but the addict in you will still panic. I like to wait about three weeks before discussing stripping the carbs from my clients' diet. As you can see from Gregory's passion for pasta, the thought of sending back the roll is anathema to most insulin-resistant people—even when they're in good blood sugar.

So. Step one is waiting till several weeks *after* you've stabilized your blood sugar.

Step two? Take the following quiz and see, once and for all, if you are a carbohydrate addict or simply a pasta lover.

▲ ▲ ▲ ▲ ▲ ▲ ▲ ▲ ▲

WHAT'S UP, DOC?

Carrots have long been the choice vegetable among dieters. They are chock-full of vitamins, minerals, and fiber. And in fact they're an appropriate hard-chew snack on my program as well. But carrots are not always as beneficial as they seem. If you're a carbohydrate addict, you might be very reactive to them—and you just might start craving carbs all over again!

The best way to find out is to go without for a few days. Then eat your carrots and see if you begin to crave more. Everyone's different, and some carbohydrate addicts can eat carrots—while others can't. Experiment. Use your judgment.

▼ ▼ ▼ ▼ ▼ ▼ ▼ ▼ ▼

ARE YOU INSULIN RESISTANT?

Note: Do not take this quiz until you've done your "five days to good blood sugar" and you've been on my diet program for at *least* two to three weeks.

See if any of the following statements are true for you. If they are, you could be a carbohydrate addict. But please, be honest. You'll still be able to eat pasta and bread. I promise.

1. Your idea of heaven is "lotsa pasta."
2. When you binge, whatever the *fathead* reason, you tend toward bread, cereal, cake, cookies, and, yes, pasta.
3. You can't stop at "one bowl."
4. A half cup of pasta to you is merely a taste. Ditto one roll, one cracker, or one slice of wholesome six-grain bread.
5. After eating carbs, you feel bloated and puffy.
6. After a carbohydrate binge, you gain weight quickly.
7. Your weight fluctuation is dramatic. You're the quintessential yo-yo dieter.
8. Although you've lost one or two pounds a week during the last month or so, you find that you've reached a plateau. You just can't lose any more weight.
9. You feel your body is more like that of the "Pillsbury Doughboy" than Linda Hamilton in *Terminator 2.*
10. You *have* to have a banana every day.
11. You can't *live* without orange juice for breakfast.
12. Whenever a colleague passes by your office, offering to get you a bagel from the coffee shop downstairs, you always say yes.
13. You always look at the desserts on a menu first.
14. You know every desk at work that has a candy jar on it.
15. You need your "chocolate bar fix" every afternoon.

16. You like to go out for drinks almost every night.
17. If the bread basket is on the table, you'll nibble without thinking.
18. Every meal has its starch.
19. You can't have a glass of wine without something to nibble, those little goldfish or peanuts or something!
20. Dessert means sugar and chocolate. You've never gotten used to the idea of fresh fruit for dessert.

If you've *passionately* answered *yes!* to any of these questions, you could very well be a carbohydrate addict. But don't despair. I have an easy way to modify my diet to meet your special needs—without sacrificing the carbs you love. I call it . . .

STRIPPING THE CARBS

Gregory sighed and settled back in the armchair. "Okay, I'm a carbo addict. I can't live without my carbs. But I still want to lose weight. What do I do?"

I smiled. "I promised you, Gregory, that my diet plan would fit into your life, that you would own it, right?"

He nodded. His mind was still on that bagel and his face had the expression "get to the point."

That's exactly what I'm going to do. Here are the rules for *stripping the carbs*. It's easy and it's painless—once you're in good blood sugar.

1. *Continue to eat your bread at breakfast.* You need the starch in the morning to maintain your blood sugar. But this literally means bread. Not rice cakes. Not cereal. Bread. (Gregory leaped at this one. He knew he couldn't eat a bagel except as a "Food You Adore," but still, six-grain bread . . . not bad.)

2. *Forgo the roll at lunch.* (Gregory shrugged. It was easy enough to ask the waiter to take the bread basket away. He could "stuff" himself on lots of grilled vegetables and some ounces of shrimp.)

3. *Contain your carbohydrates at dinner to every other day—and keep away from pasta and other highly glycemic starches, such as popcorn, bagels, white flour, and white rolls. Your good blood chemistry will maintain its balance with less reactive carbohydrates, such as winter squash or whole-grain rice.* (Okay, this one made Gregory shaky, but, after I reminded him about rice, potatoes, couscous, and lentils, even a whole-grain roll with a dab of butter, he calmed down. He remained seated.)

4. *Choose your once- or twice-a-week "Foods You Adore" from the protein or higher-fat list. Try to stay away from carbohydrate lovers' trigger foods, such as pasta, alcohol, cereal, cake, and cookies, if you possibly can. Instead think of an elaborate prime rib dinner with a baked potato and salad. A perfect Caesar salad. Peking duck. Hearty chicken vegetable soup. Even tacos and refried beans.* (Gregory liked this one. He got a faraway look in his eye and I could tell that he was ready to "give up the bagel.")

5. *Stay with this program for one week to stabilize your system. You should feel incredible, with even more energy and inner control. Your whole body will look dramatically thinner, more toned. Suddenly the pasta doesn't seem to matter at all.* (Gregory found himself rubbing his chin, checking his cheekbones. "When I was younger," he told me, "people said I looked like James Dean." James Dean or Pasta Marinara? You decide.)

6. *Once you've stabilized your* stripping the carbs *diet modification, you can take back your pasta—every third day.* But remember, a less reactive carbohydrate

is always a better choice: vegetables, whole grains, fruit. And it's always better to have your carbohydrate hits toward evening. A piece of fruit right before dinner can sometimes do the trick and you just might not want to opt for that pasta—even though it's been three days since your last plate. (And, yes, Gregory, you can have your bagel as a "Food You Adore" once a week—although it might take a little longer to get back into good blood sugar.)

7. *If you find yourself craving carbs even after three days, eat an extra apple.* Not only will you get your hard chew in and be back on the road to GBS, but because apples are both sweet and complex carbohydrate fruits, they may help satisfy your need—or they may trigger a need for more. So experiment . . . see if it works for you.

8. *Forewarned is forearmed. Don't forget to write in your food journal. Keep close tabs on your moods, your fluctuations, and your energy levels—this is crucial in* stripping the carbs. *If necessary, you might have to cut back on the pasta to every fourth day instead of every third day. Or you can use it only as an occasional "Food You Adore." It depends on how carbohydrate sensitive you are—and you can analyze that only by writing it down.* (Gregory took his journal out of his attaché case. He began to write, "Today I began to *strip the carbs*. I'm ready to look like James Dean—without the cigarette.")

DON'T SAY CHEESE

Believe it or not, both milk and cheese products contain lactose—which is a carbohydrate. If you are insulin resistant, try to restrict the cheese you eat (and of course avoid cereal and milk).

Try soy cheese, turkey, or tuna for variety. At breakfast add a slice of whole-grain bread.

❦   ❦   ❦   ❦   ❦   ❦   ❦   ❦   ❦

STRIPPING THE CARBS: THE SEQUEL

Unfortunately (or fortunately, for those more carbohydrate-sensitive than others), *stripping the carbs* is not like quitting smoking. You can't give up carbs cold turkey. First of all, you need that bread in the morning to stabilize your blood sugar. Second, carbohydrates contain important nutrients that your body needs.

So ... the best bet is to stick to those less reactive carbohydrates, the grains and the starchy vegetables, trying to have them in the evening instead of sprinkling them throughout the day. This way your body stops calling out to the insulin all day long—which only continues the cravings.

🔺   🔺   🔺   🔺   🔺   🔺   🔺   🔺   🔺

I CAN'T LIVE IN A WORLD WITHOUT BREAD

It might not be a popular tune, but it is reality for carbohydrate-addicted people—at least some of the time. Following are some tips to help you cope:

- Stay in good blood sugar. You're more sensitive to blood sugar fluctuations than non-addicts, and if you're not in good blood sugar, it's like a double whammy. There's almost nothing (except maybe Brussels sprouts) that you won't crave!
- Get the bread basket away—fast.
- Immediately order a salad so that you can crunch along with the bread eaters.
- This one's easy: Don't buy pasta, cereal, or sweet fruit when you food-shop.

- Experiment with exotic rice, beans, and lentils at dinnertime once in a while. You might even find you like it!
- On airline flights drink your water and eat your string beans—and have the stewardess take that bread/roll/cake/whatever it is away immediately.
- When dining at a friend or relative's house, have seconds on the protein and veggies. No one will even notice you haven't touched the starch. (And if they do, tell them, "Everything's delicious, but I'm stuffed, thanks." A hug is always welcome, too.)

And don't discount the fact that you "own" your diet. Experiment. Some people are more sensitive to carbohydrates than others. Perhaps you can eat a roll every third day and feel fine, whereas someone else will start hitting the cereal box as a result of that roll. *Stripping the carbs* involves some trial and error. See what carbohydrates—and when—you can handle, and adjust your diet accordingly.

I know it sounds hard right now if you are a carbohydrate addict, but here's a thought to help you along the way: You're not promising to do this forever. And why should you? You don't yet know how absolutely wonderful it feels to *strip the carbs* if you are an addict.

Remember how you felt before you did your five days on the 5-Day Miracle Diet?

And remember how incredible you felt when you finished those five days?

I make this promise—and this guarantee to all my fellow carbohydrate addicts out there: If you accurately follow my *stripping the carbs* program for three or five days, you will no longer crave that pasta with as much passion and drama as you do now.

That's all there is to it. It didn't take an entire book to

detail. I didn't tell you that pasta is bad—or that you can't eat your bread ever again.

The research regarding carbohydrate addiction is still ongoing. It's a relatively new theory, and all is not yet known about carbohydrates and particular people's resistance to insulin. But I do know one thing: It's difficult to *strip the carbs*, but if you are addicted, you will feel better and look better than you ever have in your life. It is well worth the effort.

Just think, the entire French Revolution could have ended a whole different way if the revolutionaries had only realized they could have their cake—and eat it, too!

Oh, and incidentally, I've seen Gregory for three more months now and I'd say he's more of a Brad Pitt type myself. He hasn't mentioned the *B*-word for weeks.

CHAPTER 8

Shake That Body

It's more than exercise and burning calories. When I'm walking at a fast clip, it's like food for the soul.
—*A twenty-nine-year-old male math teacher*

It's something we all know so well, it could be a mantra: exercise and diet. Exercise and diet. Exercise and diet. But clichés (or mantras) became so *because* they are so true. The fact is that exercise is crucial in *any* diet program.

And the 5-Day Miracle Diet is no exception:

"I didn't think about exercise during my five days of stabilization. If you had mentioned the word *walk* or *gym* I would have run the other way! But now? I can't wait to get on those walking shoes."

"It's weird, but being in good blood sugar actually makes me want to exercise. Me. The original couch potato!"

"Until I got in good blood sugar, the most exercise I got was walking to and from the refrigerator. Now I'll walk to the store. I'll walk down the stairs. I'll walk to a friend's house. There's no stopping me!"

"Your diet is great. But I needed to exercise to rev up my metabolism. Now I really feel alive!"

"All that extra energy has to go someplace! Why not a Stairmaster?"

These are all clients of mine, from all (excuse the pun) walks of life, from all ages and backgrounds. They know what I know: Exercise is an integral part of the 5-Day Miracle Diet. Exercise:

- Jump-starts your metabolism
- Burns calories even after you finish
- Keeps up a steady weight loss
- Helps slow down osteoporosis
- Reduces stress
- Tones your muscles
- Increases the good cholesterol (HDL) that is vital for strong, healthy hearts
- Makes you look and feel great!

So, if it's so important, why do I talk about exercise so late in the book?

WE ALL KNOW IT DOESN'T LOOK GOOD; NOW IT DOESN'T FEEL GOOD, TOO

In 1992 a fifteen-year study of over 110,000 nurses found a definite link between obesity and coronary heart disease. More recent research, as reported in *The New York Times*, has found that even moderately overweight women increase their risk of heart disease. A few years ago "middle-aged spread" was deemed okay. No more. Now women who gain over fifteen pounds after the age of eighteen almost double their risk of heart disease.

This doesn't mean we all have to look like Kate Moss, but it does mean that diet and exercise are more important than ever. And what easier way to keep the weight down than by stopping food cravings—with the 5-Day Miracle Diet.

EXERCISING YOUR OPTION

No, it's not poor organization or an oversight. The reason I don't talk about exercise way up front is the same reason I don't talk up *stripping the carbs* right away to a pasta addict. If I gave you my exercise program along with the 5-Day Miracle Diet, you'd probably run out of my office and never come back.

I don't want you to feel overwhelmed. After you've been on the 5-Day Miracle Diet for a few weeks, you'll be charged up, exuberant, ready to take on the world. *That's* when I introduce exercise. I suggest two or three days in the beginning, doing something you absolutely love. (Instead of "Food You Adore," it's "Movement You Adore" that will keep you on an exercise track.) Slowly we work up an exercise plan that consists of four to five days of both aerobic and strengthening exercises—and I haven't had a client balk yet.

Golf is the most fun you can have without taking your clothes off.

—Chi Chi Rodriguez

FEEDING THE SOUL

Joseph had been very active as a teenager and young adult. He was always the star pitcher on his Little League team; he was the captain of the basketball team in high school. Even when he was in law school, studying twenty-five hours a day, he managed to fit in a workout at the school gym before or after classes.

Something happened when he began his job in a prestigious law firm in San Diego. Perhaps it was the pressure of the job, the need to do well and stay on top. Or perhaps it was the "Welcome to the Real World" syndrome, where suddenly, abruptly, Joseph realized this was the rest of his life—and he had better earn his keep. Then again it might have been his lifestyle: power breakfasts, business lunches, and dinners with colleagues where, with a need to release tension, he'd have two or three drinks and just about anything on the menu—no matter how fat-laden and sugary it was.

I suspect it was a combination of all three. But, whatever the reason, Joseph had gained thirty-five pounds and had stopped exercising completely.

When Joseph called me to schedule an initial session during his next trip to New York, we talked a bit on the phone. I didn't discuss the diet. I simply told him to keep a food diary during the two weeks before he came to see me. I also made some minor suggestions about his lack of exercise, things such as walking up the stairs instead of taking the elevator or taking his dog for a long walk when he got home from work. I also told him to make an "appointment with himself," to actually schedule exercise, right after, say, the four o'clock meeting on Monday. That's it. Just one day. We'd worry about the rest of the week later on.

Three weeks later I saw Joseph and I explained the 5-Day Miracle Diet to him. After he got over his astonishment at its efficiency, simplicity, and logic, he smiled.

"There's something else, Adele," he said.

"Yes?"

"I organized a baseball team at my firm."

I practically leaped up from my chair, clapping with pleasure. "That's great! How did that happen?"

Joseph told me: "I took your suggestion about walking my dog. I felt guilty anyway, not spending a lot of time with him, and he's a big retriever and needs the exercise. Well, we started walking and I noticed a bunch of guys playing softball in the park. I stopped and watched."

Joseph took a sip of the water he'd brought with him. "After about ten minutes one of the guys asked me if I wanted to join them. I shook my head, but said thanks.

"I watched the whole game, remembering when I was a kid and I used to play. Suddenly I wanted to get out on that field more than anything in the world. It wasn't 'Oh, I need to exercise,' but almost a spiritual thing. Do you know what I mean?"

"Of course." I nodded. "I've been there myself."

"Well," Joseph continued, "one thing led to another and I started talking to the guys after the game. It turns out they all worked for rival law firms. That's when I got the idea. Why not us?"

Joseph now plays baseball twice a week, not because it's good for him but because he loves it. (P.S. It doesn't hurt that it's good for him, too!)

THE FRAMINGHAM STUDY

Twenty-five years ago researchers began a lon-
gitudinal study of five thousand men and women
in Framingham, Massachusetts, to see what the
risk factors for coronary heart disease were.
What they discovered—and what they continue
to discover—is that CHD is predominantly caused
by bad habits, lifestyle choices that we can change.
These include the following:

1. High blood pressure (hypertension)
2. Elevated "bad" cholesterol (LDL)
3. Cigarette smoking
4. Sedentary lifestyle
5. Stress
6. Obesity
7. Diabetes
8. Family history

Heredity certainly plays a role in developing these
risk factors. But so does environment. Learning
bad habits at an early age can contribute to your
developing these risk factors—which, incidentally,
are linked to being overweight!

There's a moral to this story—a valuable one for you
as you progress on the 5-Day Miracle Diet. In fact it's the
first principle in the exercise program I designed specifically to complement the 5-Day Miracle Diet. It's called
the Adele Excel Five-Step Exercise Plan.

ADELE EXCEL STEP 1: WE ALL KNOW THE BENEFITS OF EXERCISE, BUT UNLESS WE'RE DOING SOMETHING WE LOVE, WE'RE NOT LIKELY TO STICK WITH IT OVER THE LONG HAUL

Without even realizing it, Joseph went back to something he had loved and cherished in childhood: baseball. Think about it. When you are a child, you're one big "movement machine." You want—and need—to use those new muscles, that newfound energy, that developing curiosity. And nothing fulfills it better than play: tag, jump rope, baseball, or, as every parent knows, the ever-popular "running around and screaming at the top of your lungs" exercise.

As we get older, we forget that exercise was once fun. Suddenly it becomes something we *have* to do to stay healthy. We *have* to fit it in. No wonder we have such a difficult time!

I call exercise food for your soul. Movement inspires. Whether your passion is dance, in-line skating, or Joseph's personal choice of baseball, when you are doing exercise you enjoy, you are making your soul, not to mention your body, healthy.

So the first step in your exercise regime is finding something you love. Like the "Foods You Adore" that you eat once or twice a week, the exercise, or exercises, you choose should be picked in the spirit of fun. (And of course always check with your health professional before starting any exercise program.)

Some suggestions:

Walking

Yes, it's still a great way to get started. Anyone can do it—at any age. In fact one study of active and inactive women, at both seventy to seventy-nine years of age and nineteen to twenty years of age, found that the active seventy-year-olds more resembled the young, active nineteen-to-twenty-year-olds than they did their inactive counterparts. These women—all walkers—were more like young adults in terms of balance, strength, and flexibility than seventy-year-old senior citizens!

Walking has also been found to be a great stress reducer. A survey of over 1,700 family doctors conducted by *The Physician and SportsMedicine* found that 80 percent of primary-care doctors prescribed exercise for depression—and 60 percent prescribed it for anxiety. Their exercise of choice? An overwhelming 90 percent suggested walking.

The best way to get started is to lace up a pair of walking shoes, put on some loose, comfortable clothing appropriate for the weather, and, yes, place one foot in front of the other. That's it. Some people like to wear a Walkman or Discman while they walk; the music inspires them to greater lengths. Others listen to special walking tapes, which keep their strides within a rhythmic, timed, fat-burning pace. Still others prefer the sounds of nature, the birds in the trees, the wind whistling through the leaves, the sounds of laughter and talk. The quiet helps them solve problems at work or at home.

The Treadmill, Stairmaster, or Lifecycle Machine

Suppose it's raining. Or freezing cold. Or late at night when you shouldn't be out walking or jogging by yourself. An exercise by any other name is the exercise machine. It's convenient. You can work out anytime. You can wear whatever you want.

Many of these machines display the amount of time you're working out, the level of exertion, and the amount of calories burned. They are especially good for people who have a hard time fitting exercise into their lives. You can watch TV—and get your exercise in. You can read that proposal for work—and get your exercise in. The only drawback? A good machine can be expensive. But if it's something you'll stick with and enjoy, the machine is worth the price!

▲   ▲   ▲   ▲   ▲   ▲   ▲   ▲   ▲

A WINNING COMBINATION

Even as far back as almost twenty years ago, scientists and researchers knew that a combination of diet and exercise works best. A study done in 1979 found that a group who only dieted lost seven pounds. A group who only exercised lost six. But a third group of lucky people who both dieted and exercised lost a total of thirteen pounds!

Even more potent: After two months the diet-and-exercise group were the only ones who continued to lose weight. And guess what? Six months later it was the same story. Only a combination of diet and exercise will keep unwanted weight away for good!

▼   ▼   ▼   ▼   ▼   ▼   ▼   ▼   ▼

Exercise Videos

These are in the same category as exercise machines—with two main differences: (a) You can't watch another program while you work out; and (b) you get to look at attractive people as they go through their routines. (Men have the wider variety, from Cindy Crawford to Elle Macpherson, but women have their Lucky Luciano, and that makes up for a lot.) Exercise videos can be a lot of fun and are a good alternative when you just don't feel like going outside and walking. If you like aerobics and music with a beat, these can be great. But do choose a video that fits within your exercise level: beginner, intermediate, or advanced. And always rent before you buy. The exercise video you couldn't wait to try might turn out to be as difficult as it was for the ancient warrior Hannibal to go up the mountain with a herd of elephants.

Bicycle Riding

Although bicycles don't work those upper arms as much as walking, jogging, or aerobic exercise, there's nothing quite as exhilarating as speeding through a park, the wind whistling past you. Another plus: Bicycle riding can take you where you want to go, killing two birds with one stone, so to speak. However, *you must always wear a helmet when you ride a bicycle*.

Unless you keep to straight, smooth trails, I don't suggest bicycle riding if you have more than forty pounds to lose. It can be too strenuous on your body. Wait until you've lost five to ten pounds and give it a whirl! Until then walking is still the best policy.

Swimming

This is another good alternative to walking, especially if you belong to a gym or it's in the midst of the dog days of summer. It puts less stress on your joints, it relieves stress in your mind quite effectively, and you can do it for long periods of time without injury. However, swimming does have its drawbacks. Studies have found that you really need to swim as fast and furiously as an Olympic contender in order to burn fat—which most of us do not do. Why? When you're in water, your body sends a message to your brain, "Protect me from getting cold." The brain complies by lowering your metabolism, keeping you warmer longer.

* * *

Other "exercises for thought" include cross-country skiing, downhill skiing, in-line skating, low-impact aerobics classes, dance classes, and simply turning on the music and "letting go" in the privacy of your home.

But exercise should not only be something you absolutely enjoy, it must also be something you can do. Know your limitations. If you've been out of shape for a very long time, start slowly with walking or swimming. If you need to lose more than fifty pounds, use the treadmill on the beginner level, eventually building up your time and incline as you lose weight and get fit.

And that leads us to the second principle in the 5-Day Miracle Diet exercise regime:

ADELE EXCEL STEP 2: THINK SMALL

When Joseph decided to start playing baseball again, he didn't immediately try out for the Yankees. No, he went to the park once a week in the beginning, using those muscles and that mind-set he hadn't used since he was a child. Once a week became twice a week, then three times a week—alternated with Nautilus machines and a treadmill. This didn't happen in one month's time. It took several months to design an exercise regime he could live with, one that would not be too strenuous, that he could stick to and enjoy, and that would not send him home in a cast (or oxygen mask).

Joseph started small—and was able to increase his exercise as he became more fit. I offer the same suggestion to you: baby steps, baby steps.

Rosemary is another case in point. A successful client of mine, she was so enthusiastic to get fit and trim when she'd lost her first ten pounds that she immediately signed up for a modern-dance class in her third week on the 5-Day Miracle Diet. Wonderful—except that she hadn't taken a dance class in fifteen years and she was out of shape.

But there was Rosemary, standing in her leotards, surrounded by dancers. And I have to give her credit. One of the most common remarks I hear from my clients is that they can't go to a gym until they've lost some weight and can be "seen." Although I try to explain to them that no one's looking, I respect their choice—and I wait until they've lost more weight before I broach the subject again. But Rosemary didn't care what anybody thought. She was remarkably unself-conscious. She loved to dance and she was going to dance.

Unfortunately the body can't compensate for the mind's misperception. Rosemary saw herself as that one-time young woman in her twenties, dancing and twirling, flexible and lithe. But her body wasn't up for the exuberance. Accompanied by a rhythmic drum, Rosemary took a flying leap across the room—and landed on her ankle.

Ouch! It was several weeks before Rosemary could exercise again, and by then her enthusiasm had dampened. We needed several sessions to talk about what had happened in her modern-dance class and to come up with better exercise alternatives for the time being.

The fact is that none of us wants to feel bad. In the same way that we eventually succumb to a physiological craving, so, too, will our body call it quits if our exercise of choice is too painful. We're not going to keep something up that hurts.

Nor should exercise make us feel overwhelmed. If, like Rosemary, you do too much too soon, you might find that you simply can't keep up the pace. You become rigid, and as soon as your schedule is forced to change—whether it be a late-night meeting, a canceled date with a new person, or a sick child—you won't go back to it. Promise. It will almost feel like a relief.

No man is a failure who is enjoying life.
—William Feather

So . . . here's what I recommend on the 5-Day Miracle Diet:

- *Start with only one to three days of exercise a week, whatever you're comfortable with.* Make an appointment with yourself for those days. Write them down in your personal organizer.
- *Work up to four or five days of aerobic exercise a week* if you can—*over several months!*
- *Go for thirty minutes per workout.* It's effective and it won't tire you out. If thirty minutes at a clip is almost impossible to fit into your hectic routine, break it up. Take a ten-minute walk in the morning before you go to work. Or use your Lifecycle for ten minutes before hopping in the shower. Walk twenty minutes at lunchtime or right after work, or visit your gym for a quick aerobics class. Maybe you can even walk home from the office. Just because your activity is something you'd have to do anyway (i.e., getting from the office to your apartment) doesn't mean it doesn't qualify as exercise.

We do not stop playing because we grow old; we grow old because we stop playing.
—Anonymous

The research conclusions keep changing, but at this time many studies show that, contrary to popular belief, breaking exercise up works just as effectively as performing it at a solid clip. You'll be able to sustain a higher level of exertion because you're not tired out. And because you've taken breaks, your metabolism—the rate of which increases for one to four hours after exercise, burning additional calories and keeping energy up—will stay stronger . . . longer.

- *Use the "feel" method of exertion.* It's true that aerobic exercise is necessary to burn calories, but forget that old adage "No pain, no gain." You don't want to be so out of breath from your racewalking, for example, that you get an incredible pain in your side that makes you stop short. Nor do you want to get seriously ill from overexertion. Not only will you suffer the physical consequences but most likely you'll throw your exercise shoes into the closet and never look at them again.

On the other hand you shouldn't underdo it, either. Too little aerobic exercise and you're not burning enough calories. This means you won't lose weight as easily—and even though your body's feeling great from its good blood sugar, your metabolism will stay in the "couch-potato mode" and, more than likely, the *fathead* will rear its beastly head and try to talk you into going off the 5-Day Miracle Diet completely.

No! There is a balance between the two. It's called the target heart rate zone and it's the range within which your heart is being exercised most efficiently. The more fit you are, the more easily nutrient-rich blood can be carried to your cells—and the better able your muscles are to absorb their "food." If you're working in your target heart rate zone, you're getting the maximum results for weight loss, strong metabolism, and good health, not too much and not too little.

* * *

Great. So what is your target heart rate zone? Scientists have determined an equation, depending on how fit you are. It is based on a percentage of your maximum heart rate (MHR), or the maximum amount of times your heart beats within one minute's time. Fifty to 60 percent of your MHR is a good place for beginners to start. To lose weight, you should build up to 60 to 70 percent, eventually getting up to 80 percent after several months on the 5-Day Miracle Diet.

TARGET HEART RATE ZONE
(BEATS PER MINUTE)

Age	Target Heart Rate Zones				MHR (100%)
	50%	60%	70%	80%	
20	100	120	140	170	200
25	98	117	137	166	195
30	95	114	133	162	190
35	93	111	130	157	185
40	90	108	126	153	180
45	88	105	123	149	175
50	85	102	119	145	170
55	83	99	116	140	165
60	80	96	112	136	160
65	78	93	109	132	155

Adapted by permission from *Starting Your Personal Fitness Program* by Ann Ward, Ph.D., and James M. Rippe, M.D., Philadelphia: Lippincott-Raven Publishers, 1988, p. 10.

All well and good, but how do you know if you're in your target heart rate zone? Easy. Take your pulse while you're performing your exercise. Using a watch with a second hand, take your pulse for fifteen seconds. Multiply this number by four and you'll know how many times your heart beats per minute. If it's within your target heart rate zone, keep going. If your pulse is in a higher range, slow down a bit. Similarly, if your pulse is below your target zone, go for it . . . a little faster.

If all these scientific calculations make you feel overwhelmed (and we all know what happens if you begin to feel overwhelmed!), there's an easier way. I call it the "feel" method of exertion. If you are doing aerobic exercise and you can feel your heart pumping, so far so good. If you can also carry on a conversation while you're exercising, then most likely you are in your target heart rate zone and doing just fine. If you can't talk because you're out of breath, slow down! If you can not only talk but sing a rock 'n' roll song, go faster!

PULSE POINTS

You need to know how to take your own pulse if you're going to determine your target heart rate zone.

1. The most common place to take your pulse is just inside your wrist bone. Use your second and third fingers. *Never* use your thumb; it has its own beat.
2. Some people have soft arteries at their wrists and cannot feel a pulse. Don't worry! You're not dead. Try your neck's carotid artery, the area right below each ear and beside the jawline.
3. If you have difficulty finding your pulse there, try placing your fingers at your temple, right above your brow bone, or at the side of your Adam's apple.
4. Remember to time the beats for fifteen seconds, then multiply by four to get a reading. Practice a few times before you exercise so that your natural flow and enjoyment aren't interrupted!

In other words you want strenuous, but not overly so.

For me the "feel" method is best. When a client's weight loss slows down and all other avenues are explored, I'll recommend he become more exact in his exercise program to determine if he is getting the maximum benefits. Otherwise feel, enjoy, have fun!

NO, IT'S NOT A NEW ON-LINE CODE

VO2 Max is the maximum oxygen consumption your body can handle. Our bodies need oxygen so that we can live. Period.

But the more fit you are, the better and more efficient your body is at getting that oxygen through your entire system. If you exercise at 60 to 70 percent of your VO2 Max, you will improve your heart's capability in pumping blood through your body and you can better help your muscles extract necessary oxygen from this blood—all of which translates into more energy.

Increase your heart's ability to pump oxygen-rich blood to those hungry muscles and the result is fitness. You can garden, shovel the snow, run up the stairs, and jump on a bus with much more ease and finesse.

How do you know if you're exercising at 60 or 70 percent of your VO2 Max? Easy. Either use your target heart rate zone chart and check your pulse or use the old standby, levels of exertion. If it feels strenuous but not overly so, you're doing great. And, yes, even walking for short intervals has been found to increase VO2 Max in people of all ages and at all fitness levels.

ADELE EXCEL STEP 3: MIX TONING
EXERCISES WITH AEROBIC EXERCISES

Even if Joseph could play baseball every night of the week, he'd shake his head no—and it has nothing to do with his hectic schedule. After three months on the 5-Day Miracle Diet, Joseph knows something that a lot of people don't: As I mentioned to him, research studies have recently shown that aerobic exercise is great, but it must be tempered with resistance strength-training exercises.

I remember going to a gym about ten years ago. It held continuous low-impact aerobics classes, with an occasional yoga class sprinkled in. However, even these few and far between yoga classes were dropped because no one attended (except for me and a few enlightened others). The reason? Everyone wanted to burn calories, to lose weight, and get muscular. And somehow the word got out that you had to sweat to get these benefits.

Even the scientific community agreed. In the old days (about three years ago) studies reported that only aerobic exercise was necessary to lose weight—the more stomping and running and jumping the better. After all, *aerobic* literally means "in the presence of air." Oxygen is pumped through our system; our muscles work out, getting strong with a continuous supply of nutrient-pumping blood. Calories are burned, and stored fat in the cells are used up. With these kinds of credentials it's no wonder that aerobic exercise has its own place on the fitness pedestal.

Anaerobic exercise, on the other hand, only burns a few calories. Weight lifting. Nautilus machines. Yoga. In these and other exercises energy is sustained in two- or three-minute intervals only. You don't have to bother taking your pulse to know you're not anywhere near your target heart rate zone.

However, anaerobic, or resistance strength-training exercise, has other things going for it. Strengthening and toning are the only proven ways to increase lean muscle tissue—which translates into slimmer stomachs, trimmer thighs, and broader chests. Strengthening and toning exercises also improve your posture and reduce stress.

Ideally I like everyone on the 5-Day Miracle Diet to eventually spend three days a week on aerobic exercise and two alternate days on strength and toning exercises. Research conclusions are always changing and this, too, might have a different face in a year or two. But for now, it's safe to say, strengthen and walk, lift weights and run, take a yoga class and a low-impact aerobics one. And don't forget, if you're doing something you love, you will *want* to get out there and "just do it!"

In the same way that good blood sugar continues to stop those omnipotent cravings, so, too, does exercise feed on itself. The more you do it, the more you want to do it. Feeling fit and healthy. There's nothing like it in the world!

Some good strengthening and toning exercises include the following:

- Yoga
- Toning classes and exercises that pinpoint various parts of the body: upper arms, waist and back, stomach, thighs, legs, and buttocks
- Weight resistance machines, such as Nautilus and Bailey
- Weight lifting
- T'ai chi, kung fu, and karate classes
- Stretch classes and exercises
- Ballet classes

ADELE EXCEL STEP 4: PLAN STRATEGIES
TO FIT EXERCISE INTO YOUR LIFE

It was easy for Joseph to plan baseball games. He loved it! So he simply made an appointment with himself and wrote it down in his book:

Thursday nights—baseball in the park
Sunday A.M.—baseball in the park

That took care of his baseball games, but what about the other five days in the week?

Writing down the times you plan to exercise can help you stick to it. There it is in black and white (or on your computer screen): exercise class at lunch, meet J. and walk after work, yoga Saturday afternoon.

You wouldn't miss a meeting or an important dinner if it was written in your book. Chances are you won't miss your exercise appointments, either.

I suggested some other strategies to Joseph to get him to keep to his exercise regime. To recap:

- Try listening to a book on tape while you walk, jog, or use a Lifecycle machine. You'll be so busy wondering what happens next that you'll forget that you're exercising—and as with a great soap opera, you will be counting the hours until your next session!
- Do exercise that's not really exercise: Walk past your destination and back again. Park ten blocks farther away from your office building. Use the stairs instead of the elevator. Take the dog for a longer walk. Get off your bus or train two stops before or after your regular one. Remember, exercise can be broken up into segments; you will still get the same benefits as if you were concentrating on your jumps in front of your

health club's mirror. And you'll be surprised at how these "exercise quickies" can add up . . . to a solid thirty minutes of aerobics!

- Remember the "six-month rule." Studies show that if you keep something up for six months, it becomes a habit. Even if you stop exercising after six months for whatever reason, you'll eventually come back to it because it's been ingrained in your routine.

- Try the buddy system. Working out with a friend really does help. After all, if you're supposed to meet someone for a jog around the park, you'd hate to disappoint him or her. Cancellations can cause friction between friends—not to mention extra pounds! Further, a friend is there when you just don't feel up to exercising. He or she can push you, cajole you, or simply tell you to get up and get moving! Support is a wonderful thing.

- Keep in mind that the most difficult part of exercising is getting up to do it. Once you're out the door with your exercise gear, you've won the battle!

- Variety is the spice of life. If possible, find a few exercises you love. Perhaps, in a given week, you'll take a jazz-dance class, a walk in the mall, two days of Lifecycle, two days of yoga, and an aqua aerobics class. With that kind of schedule, there's no time to be bored.

  If consistency is important to you, however, don't deviate too much. You'll feel overwhelmed. If you like the idea of hopping out of bed and getting out the door for a walk every morning at six o'clock, don't stop. But do try a different route every so often. Use a treadmill. Go to the health club and watch people as you walk around the track. Change the music or book you are listening to on your Walkman.

- Reward yourself! Like the 5-Day Miracle Diet, nonfood rewards are essential for keeping the *fathead* at bay and keeping you on track. The exercise *"lazyhead"* might not be as deadly as the blood sugar's *fathead*, but it can still push a onetime couch potato back into the sack.

To avoid greeting the *lazyhead*, attack it head-on—with a reward to keep you moving. These can be the same rewards as for your diet plan: A ticket to a tennis match. A movie. A massage. A facial. A haircut. And, to combine the two, how about a weekend or at least a day at a nearby spa? You'll not only eat right, but you'll get great exercise in a beautiful, stress-reducing setting.

FIRST THINGS FIRST

Warmups and cooldowns are not the parts you fast-forward on your video or on your Sony Walkman. They are crucial components to any exercise program, preventing injury and keeping flexibility high.

Warmups can be whatever activity you plan to do—only done at a slower pace—for five minutes. This means strolling if you're going to walk or jog, or simply waltzing around the room if you're going to rock 'n' roll.

Cooldowns help you relax. They are simple stretches. You can do all or any portion of my fifteen-minute stretch after your exercise session—or simply slow down. Go back to that stroll or that slow dance for five minutes.

One important note: *Never, ever* do any stretches, strengthening, or toning exercises without first warming up. And when you are finished with your stomach curls, your push-ups, and your free weights, don't forget the cooldown, too.

ADELE'S EXCEL STEP 5: DO MY FIFTEEN-MINUTE
STRETCH WHENEVER YOU WANT TO FEEL GREAT!

In the same way that I developed my ideas about diet, I went about developing a specific exercise that would not only tone the body, keep heart rates up, and reduce stress but would also have people coming back to it again and again.

I used myself, the original *lazyhead*. I figured that if I could devise an exercise program that I actually looked forward to, then *everyone* would want to do it! So, over the years, as I researched blood sugar and hormonal secretions, I also researched metabolism and muscle mass. I studied yoga, t'ai chi, and other alternative exercise regimes. I also jogged mile after mile to see what it would do for my body and my mind.

The result? My unique fifteen-minute stretch that not only uses every part of the body, but energizes you while reducing stress. It's great for toning and it's great for burning. You don't need any unusual equipment, just some loose-fitting clothes and a comfortable, private area in which to do the stretches. An exercise mat or a heavy, folded blanket on a hardwood floor or carpet is fine (a plain hardwood floor is a bit too hard); even if your feet stick out over the edge, you'll still have a feeling of containment and security. (Some of your favorite soothing music helps, too, for atmosphere: jazz, New Age, ballads, whatever you like.)

A few of the exercises require two tennis balls stuffed into the bottom of a sock. If you assemble this beforehand, you won't have to interrupt the flow of your fifteen-minute stretch.

When you have finished this stretch, you will have nurtured yourself without food. You will also feel great—and people will notice a positive change in your body as time goes by. The best part? It takes only fifteen minutes. You can do it anytime you want, any day and anywhere. I've been known to do my fifteen-minute stretch two times in one day—and so have several of my clients. (Even Joseph, the baseball dreamer, has used my fifteen-minute stretch before an important meeting.) *One note: Don't do this stretch without warming up. Take a warm shower if you've just gotten up. Walk the dog. Anything, as long as you've moved around some and have warmed up.*

So . . . what are we waiting for! Here it is, step by step, my fifteen-minute rejuvenating routine. Read it through once so that you understand it. Remember, it might take several times before you know it by heart. Don't be discouraged. Just tote this book with you and leave it open to this page! (*And, as always, please show this stretch to your health professional before beginning this or any exercise program.*)

The 5-Day Miracle Diet Fifteen-Minute Stretch

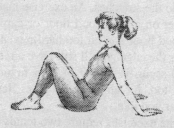

1. Begin by sitting on the floor, feet flat in front of you, about twelve inches away from your body or whatever is comfortable. Lean back on your arms, palms flat on the floor, taking the tension off your back. This will also relax your leg muscles a bit.

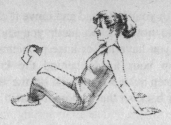

2. Allow your knees to move slowly to the right, then to the left, back and forth, as you're rolling on the large muscle mass of your buttocks, the area located between the large hip joints. Remember: no pushing or straining, just a natural falling from side to side, your knees moving to the distance that is comfortable.

As you gently roll your knees from side to side a few times, you'll notice that by rolling on the large muscles of your buttocks, you are actually moving these muscles—the area where so many of us hold lots of tension!

Focus on how you feel. Sore? Tight? Tense? Comfortable? This exercise is a self-massage; the gentle rocking on your tension points soothes and relaxes them. Rock on tender spots if you wish. Feel those sore areas disappear.

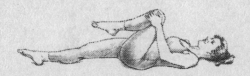

3. Lie down gently on your back. Take two or three deep breaths. Feel yourself unwinding. Bring your left leg up off the floor, bending it at the knee. Slowly move it toward your chest. Clasp your knee

gently with your left hand and move it closer to your chest. (Do not pull too hard; you should feel no pain!) If you have hip or knee problems or discomfort, clasp your hands behind the knee, making sure to keep your lower back on the floor. Do not arch your back so that abdominals will then also be engaged.

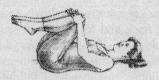

4. Now, still clasping your left knee, gently bring your right leg up, bending it at the knee. Slowly move it toward your chest. Clasp your right knee gently with your right hand and move it closer to your chest. (Remember, no pain!)
5. Let your right knee fall slowly to the right and just as you feel a slight pulling in your groin as if your left leg wants to follow, allow it to do so. Rest with your bent right leg on the floor and your bent left leg on top. Breathe!

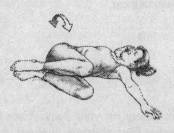

6. Reverse the movement, slowly rolling your left knee to the left, your right leg following. Do this right-left

roll slowly four or five times. Feel how it massages your lower back as it gently stretches your inner thighs and groin. Work up to ten rolls, knowing that with each roll you are giving your body an opportunity to stretch muscles, lubricate joints, and ease tension. Breathe deeply and naturally. You should experience a feeling of letting go. (As you get in better condition and you feel more flexible, you may take your hands off your knees and place your arms outstretched on the floor.) As you lead with your bent leg and follow with the other to a resting position (leg on top), you will create a wonderful twisting stretch. You should feel a gentle pull only. Perform four to five times. Slowly build up to ten repetitions. Remember to keep breathing as you exercise. Relax. If you feel any pain, stop! Be careful not to exceed your body's limitations. (Adapted from the Feldenkrais Method.)

7. Let your legs roll back on the floor. Lie back on the floor using your arms to support the movements. Pull your knees to your chest. Now that you've warmed up, you should be able to more easily clasp your hands around your legs at knee level or behind your knees. Hug your knees as tightly as you can to your chest. If you are in good condition, clasp each hand at the wrist with the other hand and hug your legs at the shin.

8. With your hands still clasped around your bent knees, rock in whatever direction feels comfortable, either right to left or back to front. Rocking is a very primal movement; it can be very soothing. Breathe deeply two or three times, in and out, in and out, in and out. Slowly. Feel the massage on your lower back. Stop if you feel any discomfort.

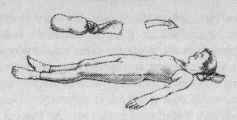

9. Still lying on the floor, put your tennis-ball sock behind your neck, just underneath the occipital bones
   (the two bones at the base of your skull). Adjust
   yourself to find a comfortable resting place with the
   tennis-ball sock supporting the weight of your head
   completely. Relax. Breathe deeply two or three
   times. Let go. Ah. That's it.
10. Remove your tennis-ball sock. Use your fingers (pri-
    marily your thumbs and forefingers) to gently mas-
    sage the same area. Take the time to notice any sore
    spots and massage these areas a little longer.
11. Now sit up slowly on your knees, if you can, heels up
    and under your buttocks, back straight. (If you have
    knee pain or any other limiting factors, do this exercise
    in a standing position.) Clasp your hands on top of your
    head, then push them toward the ceiling, palms up.
    Move slightly from side to side. Feel a good stretch in
    your upper arms and the sides of your body!

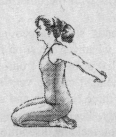

12. Still sitting tall and straight on your knees (or standing, if you need to), clasp your hands behind your lower back. Gently raise them behind you until you feel a gentle stretch in your arms, shoulders, and upper torso. Be careful not to arch your back. Breathe in deeply to a count of four, then breathe out to a count of four. Perform this twice slowly.

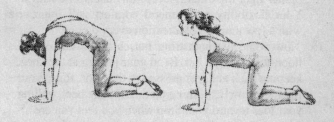

13. Now that the large muscles in your legs, chest, buttocks, neck, and arms are stretched, it's time to do the cat and dog stretch. Get on your hands and knees. Drop your head down. Breathe in and as you exhale, tuck your stomach in while curving your back toward the ceiling. Count to five. Then let your body go. Inhale and let your stomach relax, while arching your back and bringing your head up in the same move. Repeat three times.

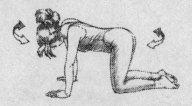

14. Next, still in the same position, try moving your head from side to side while you "wag your tail."

You can either move your head and your buttocks in the same direction, first left, then right, or you can try opposite sides, head to the left, buttocks to the right. Then, head to the right, buttocks to the left. The possibilities are endless—as long as you are feeling a good stretch. There is no right or wrong. Do what feels good for you. It's natural for one side to be tighter than the other. Accept this and work with it. Your flexibility and general comfort will improve with a few minutes of attention every day.

15. Now come the hamstring muscles: Lie flat on the floor, legs straight out. Bend your left leg at the knee, keeping back and feet pressed to the floor. Raise your right leg slowly, pushing up through the heel, pulling your toes toward you. Stop when you feel you are almost to your limit. Breathe! (You can use a belt with this stretch: Put it around the ball of the foot of your raised leg and hold the belt with your hands.) Always keep your head and shoulders on the floor. To stretch these muscles properly, your movement needs to be long and slow. Take three breaths and count slowly while your leg is raised.

Alternate legs, repeating three times on each leg. And accept your limitations. They will change with time!

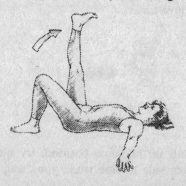

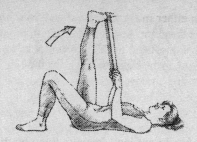

16. Still on your back, stretch your left leg out on the floor. Using your clasped hands or your belt, pull your right knee toward your right armpit/torso area. Feel the groin get stretched. Hold for a count of four. *Breathe!* Repeat three times on each side.

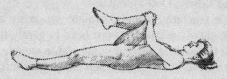

17. Lie back on the floor. Close your eyes. Pull all your muscles tight. Make a fist. Crinkle your toes. Scrunch your neck. Pull in your stomach. Squeeze your eyes shut. Grimace. Inhale and hold for a count of four. Then exhale and relax, letting everything go—your eyes, your stomach, your mouth, your arms, and your legs. Take four deep breaths, your eyes closed.

18. With your eyes closed and your body relaxed, take a minute to move in any way that your body seems to want to. Roll your head from side to side. Or draw your bent knees up again and rock from side to side. Or roll your entire body onto one side, then the other. Or just allow yourself to be, for a moment, just the way you are.

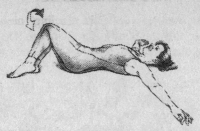

19. Slowly bend your legs, keeping them on the ground. Slowly move your bent legs toward your torso, rolling your body gently from side to side.
20. Now use your arms to help lift your upper torso into a sitting, cross-legged position. Allow your head to hang forward. Breathing deeply, slowly lift your head.
21. Stand slowly. Don't jump up!
22. When you are standing straight up, arms at your sides, slowly allow just your head to gently tilt over the left shoulder. Feel a comfortable stretch on the right side as you lean your left ear to your left shoulder. Now tilt your head to the right shoulder. Feel a comfortable stretch on the left side as you tilt your head to the right. Remember not to bend at the waist.

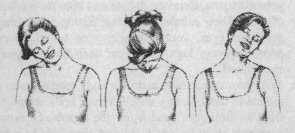

23. Still standing, gently roll your head in a circle, beginning with a tilt to the left, your left ear toward your left shoulder. Then tilt your head down to your

chest in front of you. Still circling, now tilt your right ear toward your right shoulder. Do this two times in one direction, then two times in the opposite direction.

24. Close your eyes. Move your head back to center. Take a deep breath in through your nose, your mouth closed, to the count of four. Then slowly exhale through your mouth, again to the count of four. Repeat. Open your eyes.

25. That's it! You should feel relaxed, toned, and ready to face whatever lies ahead—from a *fathead* situation to a delightful evening out that includes a "Food You Adore"!

There's only one thing left to share: some of the common questions I've encountered among my thousands of clients. Once your questions are answered, you'll be ready not only to begin the rest of your life but to begin a whole *new*, exhilarating life as well!

CHAPTER 9

"What Is Food Suicide?" and Other Questions My Clients Ask

What makes this diet different, what really makes it different for me, is the fact that it is so simple. I mean, my biggest question is, "Why don't I have more *questions?"*

—*A fifty-three-year-old magazine editor*

Congratulations! You now have the complete 5-Day Miracle Diet at your fingertips. You know—and own—the diet. You understand the chemistry behind food cravings—and the psychological *fatheads* that sometimes get in the way. You know the value of exercise and you can now see how it can easily fit into your day—especially with my fifteen-minute stretch.

Now that you have the knowledge, there's only one thing left. And that's to do it!

THE NEXT QUESTION, PLEASE

As you start feeling better than you ever have in your entire life, you might come across some questions, some things you're just not sure of. This chapter is designed to help you through some of those questions.

The more you learn, the more you want to learn. The more knowledge you have, the more you need to know.

My clients are no exception. As they embark on their exciting new lives, the questions always crop up. From Joseph to Charlotte, from Bonnee to Jack, from Donna to Arthur, from Rosemary to the thousands of other clients who have come through my office doors—all of them have had questions they needed answered. And despite the different ages, the different social strata, the different issues surrounding their weight, there are always some questions that come up again and again.

Based on the questions they have asked, I've constructed the following questions and answers, some very general, some more specific, to help all of you, the readers out there who can't come to my office, understand, stay with, and enjoy life on the 5-Day Miracle Diet.

"What Is Food Suicide?"

No, it is not death by eating, but it is a very self-destructive act. There you are, in good blood sugar, your physiological cravings gone for good, then, suddenly, you find yourself looking at that croissant or that tortellini or that apple tart. You distract yourself. You identify the problem and recognize what you can do about it. Perhaps it's the fact that you're meeting your new in-laws for the first time. Perhaps it's the criticism you got at work from your boss. Perhaps it's the fight you just had with a close friend.

Whatever it is, you know it's the *fathead* at work—and you know what to do about it. You can distract yourself. You can eat some carrots. You can go for a massage. You can rent a movie.

But you don't. Instead you listen to that inner saboteur, that destructive inner whisper that says, "Fail. You don't deserve to look and feel great. Fail."

You're on the fence. You want to succeed and yet you feel such pressure in your life. A deeply hidden part of you secretly believes you don't deserve it. Somewhere, deep inside, is a sense of self-loathing.

So what do you do? You don't binge because, after all, you are in good blood sugar and 90 percent of your mind-set wants to keep going strong. On the other hand, that 10 percent of *fathead* sabotage is talking, and getting stronger every day. You can't resist completely.

Instead you tease yourself. Maybe you eat a soft chew in the morning instead of the afternoon. Maybe you decide to have a pasta dish at lunch. Maybe you eat a frozen yogurt instead of dinner.

Get the picture? You're eating just enough to keep your chemistry continually off balance—and your craving strong. Eventually you'll succumb to those cravings. You won't be able to help it. Thanks to the *fathead,* your physiological component of the 5-Day Miracle Diet is heading for a bad-blood-sugar nosedive.

Like any other bad habit, from cigarettes and alcohol to eating high-fat foods if you have high cholesterol, this form of suicide will eventually kill—if not yourself, at least your 5-Day Miracle Diet and all the wonderful things that go along with it.

"If I Am Eating a Late Dinner, Should I Eat a Late Lunch So That I Won't Get Hungry Later?"

Even though it seems so logical to agree, believe it or not, the answer to this one is no. Contrary to popular belief, if you are having a late dinner, it is even *more* important to eat your lunch and your snacks on time. This will maintain your good blood sugar—which in turn will keep you from craving that bread basket or fattening entrée at dinner. Instead of a late lunch have an extra hard- or soft-chew snack—or snacks—in the afternoon at appropriately timed intervals.

"What About Dairy Products?"

If you eat enough of the calcium-rich food on my program and take a calcium supplement at night, you should be getting enough calcium in your diet so that you won't need excessive amounts of dairy products. However, I am not against a glass of skim milk, some cottage cheese, or an occasional slice of cheese. If you really like your dairy, have that glass of skim or 1% milk once a day.

One vital point, actually two, and they are called *lactase* and *lactose*. Lactase is a digestive enzyme produced by the body. Lactose is the sugar found in milk products that can create gassiness, heartburn, and a bloated feeling—if people don't have enough of the right enzyme (lactase) to digest it. Lactose can be highly reactive. If you are insulin-resistant, the carbohydrates in the milk can set off a craving. The trigger comes from what lactose is composed of: sugar. Like other sugars, lactose is easily broken down in your system. Insulin is rushed to the scene and . . . the rest is blood-sugar history.

If you're not insulin-resistant, no problem. The insulin does its job and the broken-down lactose goes to feed your waiting cells. But if you are sensitive, watch out! Like certain carbohydrates (which break down into different sugars for the cells' food), milk products are highly glycemic and the insulin rushes in, does its job, and hangs out waiting for more. Like pasta and other highly glycemic carbohydrates, milk can be dangerous to your good-blood-sugar health, creating havoc in your system and jettisoning a chemical imbalance.

If you feel bloated, gassy, or experience heartburn after consuming a dairy product, you could be lactose-intolerant. A better bet? Get your calcium from the other foods in the 5-Day Miracle Diet and, if you must drink milk, try one of the new lactose-free skim-milk products.

"When I Get Up Late on a Weekend, Should I Just Skip Breakfast?"

No! Whether you rise early or late, all your body knows is that it has not received food for quite a long time. Your blood sugar has been dropping while you've been having sweet dreams. It now needs correcting—fast. That's why you must eat breakfast within a half hour (or three-quarters of an hour, if you're exercising) of waking up—whatever time that is. Eat lunch within two hours of starting breakfast, followed by a hard-chew snack every two hours. (After the first hard-chew snack, the others can be soft-chew snacks.) Plan to eat dinner no later than seven o'clock. Adapting your GBS schedule to a late-morning weekend will help stabilize your blood sugar—especially if you end up with your last meal around the same time as always.

"I Thought Insulin Had to Do with Diabetes, not Cravings. Isn't That Still True?"

Insulin has everything to do with diabetes. I have never discounted that on my 5-Day Miracle Diet. However, it is my belief that late-onset diabetes *starts* with years of bad-blood-sugar abuse. The excess insulin that is manufactured in a bad-blood-sugar state creates an imbalance that leads not only to obesity, fatigue, poor concentration, and moodiness but eventually to such physical ailments as late-onset diabetes. The insulin that is produced works too hard to try to keep your blood-sugar levels even, a battle it cannot win. Eventually the consistently high insulin levels can result in late-onset (or Type II) diabetes, which is a condition in which the cells become resistant to insulin or not enough insulin is produced to lower blood-sugar levels. All the more reason to be in GBS now! It's never too late.

"I Overate Last Night, So, to Compensate, Today I Skipped the Bread with Breakfast. Is This Okay?"

If only we could erase the mistakes of yesterday! We'd all be skinny, kind, and never without a day of exercise. Unfortunately there's no such thing as compensation. If you overate in one meal, you can't make up for it by eating less at another. The 5-Day Miracle Diet doesn't work that way. Remember, the whole key to my program is controlled blood sugar. The only way to raise and maintain good blood sugar is to eat the foods I suggest at the times and in the combinations I carefully spell out. If you miss your bread at breakfast today, you'll be in even worse blood sugar than you were last night when you overate. The best plan of action? Pick yourself up, dust yourself off, and start fresh with a GBS-appropriate breakfast within a half hour of waking up.

"How Do I Maintain My Weight Without Gaining Back Any of My Hard-Lost Pounds?"

By the time you've lost as much weight as you want to on the 5-Day Miracle Diet, I would be confident to say you own the program as much as Danny, Charlotte, Bonnee, or even me! You have learned how to eat, at what times and in what combinations. You have learned to travel with your program, work with your program, go out to dinner with your program. You have the "Foods You Adore" when you want them—and only in the amounts that satisfy. You have faced the *fathead* head-on and you can identify and recognize what your sabotaging issues are. In fact you feel absolutely fabulous almost 100 percent of the time!

Like life itself, the 5-Day Miracle Diet is dynamic. It is always changing, always bending, with you and your needs, your wishes, and your lifestyle. If you follow the maintenance program I've outlined for you in this book, you don't have to worry. Relax! Remember, the weight-loss segment of the plan is really a practice session for maintenance. The work has been done for you. If you continue to lose weight, add an extra fruit or protein. If you start gaining weight, cut back on that extra portion. Measure your food again to make sure you are eyeballing correctly. Examine your food diary. Are you exercising enough? Are you drinking your water?

Remember, you are in control. You can analyze your unique situation and handle it. You can be in good blood sugar for the rest of your life—and enjoy every single moment of it!

"Help! I'm Beginning to Crave My Trigger Food! What Do I Do?"

Cindy came to see me in a panic one afternoon. She looked like a nervous wreck.

"Cindy! What's the matter?" I asked.

"I'm in trouble, Adele. Big trouble."

After "shooting the scale"—and discovering she'd lost two pounds—Cindy sat down.

"So what's going on, Cindy?" I asked. "You lost two more pounds. You should be delighted. Instead you're extremely upset. Tell me, please, what's the matter?"

Cindy took a deep breath. "It's the brownies at my corner bakery. They're beautiful. Big, fat squares with walnuts and dark icing. I keep thinking about them. For three days I've thought about them. I can't work. I can't carry on a conversation. I want a brownie! In fact as soon as I left here, I planned on going home and getting a half dozen. After all, I already got weighed for the week."

Cindy's situation is very common. There you are, in good blood sugar, feeling great and losing weight, and boom! The brownie/cookie/ice cream/chocolate/pasta cries out, "Eat me . . . eat me."

First things first: Check over your food diary. Any forgotten hard chews? Any middle-of-the-afternoon pastas? Any delayed snacks or lunchtimes? If all looks good, it means your chemistry is in good shape—and you are still in good blood sugar. It can be several days of near misses rather than one large binge.

The problem? Obviously it's the *fathead* at work. Think about your current situation. Are things stressful at home or work? Is there an event coming up that might be making you nervous? For Cindy the problem was two-fold. Her ex-husband was getting married the following week, and a good friend of both of them was attending. And at work the CEO of her company was coming for several days to chat with every manager one-on-one.

It would make anyone want a brownie!

The best solution? Once Cindy identified her *fathead* issues, she could do one of many things: She could give herself a nonfood reward; she could relieve her nervousness and, yes, her jealousy, by speaking with a supportive friend or simply writing her feelings down. Or, if the emotional hunger is so strong that even these *fathead* weapons don't work, Cindy can use the delay technique, eating some carrots while telling herself she can have the brownie if she really needs it afterward. She can distract herself with a magazine or yet another call. But if time passes and all else fails, she should march into the bakery, head high, order one brownie and have as little as possible to satisfy her need as the "Food You Adore" portion of her 5-Day Miracle Diet. And, most important, she should keep going strong.

Identify and recognize. That's all there is to it. The next time a craving calls out, simply say hello. You don't have to stop and chat.

"I'm Bored! What Can I Do?"

Boredom is a double-edged sword. On one edge, there's the blood-sugar enemy. If you are teasing your body with wrong scheduling or snacks, you could be in bad blood sugar, which causes cravings—which in turn makes you feel bored. You might also be coming back from a night of "Food You Adore"—especially if you drank more than usual and ate more sugar than you normally do. Until your chemistry is back in shape, you might experience cravings here and there for up to forty-eight hours— which might translate into a sensation of feeling bored with your food. Fill those "coming back" hours with non-food nourishment: a massage. Shopping. A tennis game. Use your emotional "food" to distract and desist.

The other edge of boredom's sword holds the *fathead* enemy. Perhaps you've been eating the same foods day in and day out on purpose, unconsciously sabotaging yourself so that you'll get bored and drop out. Or perhaps it isn't an unconscious sabotage. Maybe you genuinely love a slice of bread with no-fat cheese. But after four weeks enough might be enough. Experiment! Live a little! Try some turkey for breakfast. Tofu with mustard (Yes, it really is delicious!) on a rice cake. An egg. Or unsweetened cereal with skim milk (on alternate days).

There's enough food on this program to stop boredom in its tracks—if that's what you want. Remember, just as food doesn't have to be the "weapon of choice," so, too, can boredom be kept at bay.

"I'm Going to a Friend's House for Dinner—and She's Made a Special (Fattening) Dish Especially for Me. Help!"

I can't tell you how often I've heard this refrain. But I have one of my own that makes for perfect "harmony":

compliment, compliment, compliment. Whether it's an "other-people's food" sabotage at work or simply ignorance, it doesn't matter. You can counterattack. What is your friend saying with her special dish? Think about it. She's saying, "I love you. I want you to know how special you are to me. That's why I made this dish."

It goes deeper. She also might be saying, "Do you love me, too?"

That's why a compliment works so well. A hug and a passionate, but honest refrain: "You are a wonderful cook and I feel absolutely perfect. Everything was fabulous. I love you for doing all this! In fact I feel so perfect that I just want to sit here for a while. I want the moment to last."

Then you can go on with one of the following:

- "I'm so stuffed. I'll eat some later, promise." (Everyone will forget about it.)
- "I love you for this and I'll take some home. But I'm on a diet and I'm feeling really good about it now." (Friends should understand.)
- "I'd love some." (Then you mix it with the other food on your plate or take one small bite.)
- If it is indeed something you like, then make it a "Food You Adore" and eat as much as *you* need to feel satisfied—not as much as you think your friend needs for you to eat! And of course enjoy every morsel!

"How Do I Know When to Stop Losing Weight?"

This is an individual question—with an individual answer. When Bonnee lost twenty-five pounds, she discovered that her clothes were now much looser. She liked what she saw in the mirror when she was dressed. "Even my pantyhose are more comfortable!" she told me with glee.

Bonnee was ready to maintain her weight, not lose any more. She felt terrific. She had a tremendous amount of energy. And she was completely confident of her looks and style. There was no reason to lose more weight.

Jack, on the other hand, had lost thirty pounds, but he still hated the way he looked in his jeans. He was tired of buying "he-man" pants and shirts. His blood pressure was still high. He wanted to lose another twenty pounds—and it seemed reasonable. To keep his *fathead* at bay, he began to exercise four days a week instead of three. He experimented with different foods. He made it a point to go out to the movies and see every new release—feeding his emotional hunger instead of his belly. In Jack's case he was entirely in the right to want to lose more weight. And who knows? Maybe when he lost another ten, he'd feel enough was enough, even though he'd originally said twenty.

In other words the numbers on the scale don't mean anything. They are just guidelines as you continue on your 5-Day Miracle Diet. What does matter is how you look and feel. It's not about looking in the mirror when you're completely naked and noticing every bump and fold. It's about walking down the street and seeing yourself in a storefront reflection.

"Wow! That's me. I feel great!"

That's all you need to say (to yourself or to someone close) to know when to stop losing weight.

"What Are Your Feelings About Alternative Therapies?"

I've never liked the word *alternative*. It implies that there is a different, almost "weird" way of healing than taking pills and getting tests. Ask a billion Chinese whether acupuncture is alternative and they'll give you a puzzled look. Similarly, herbs and teas are still used in the East—

and in Europe—as much as they were thousands of years ago, long before antibiotics and X rays. Even the royal family of England consults a homeopathic physician. "Alternative" therapies include the obvious ones, such as nutrition, diet, and exercise—all of which are a part of the 5-Day Miracle Diet—as well as the less obvious and less conventional modalities, such as:

- Homeopathy
- Massage
- Natural vitamins
- Aromatherapy
- Herbology
- Acupuncture
- Meditation and creative visualization
- Yoga
- Bach flower remedies

However, the scientist in me also has an important respect for scientific technology. Many of the ailments of today's modern world would not be cured were it not for the advances made in standard medicine.

As with most things, a synergistic combination of the two points of view makes for a healthy, productive life. "Alternative" therapies focus on wellness, on preventing disease before it occurs. They concentrate on nutrition and diet, exercise, and stress-reducing techniques. Standard medicine focuses on containing the disease once it is in place.

Both of these have their place. Preventive medicine, with its emphasis on alternative methodologies, will help stop disease from taking root. But illness is complicated, and there are so many variables as to why people get sick, from genetic to accidental, so, when something serious strikes, it would be irresponsible not to see a physician to get a complete examination and a professional diagnosis.

"How Do I Modify My Diet If I'm Going on a Plane in Different Time Zones?"

Here's another plus for the 5-Day Miracle Diet. If you happen to be a frequent flyer, whether for business or for pleasure, my program will help tremendously in preventing jet lag. A state of good blood sugar keeps your energy up and your hormones on an even keel. And by eating planned snacks and meals on time, you're keeping a steady, calm internal clock.

A few tips:

Always eat breakfast before boarding the plane. You never know when those little trays will come around, and it's vital that you eat on time. And lest you forget, salted nuts and itty-bitty pastries, sandwiches, and crackers are not good food choices. Let's face it, who would want to waste a "Food You Adore" on an airline's "Salisbury steak"?

A good counterattack to the plastic menus also includes BYOS (bring your own snacks). Baby carrots. Cut-up cabbage. Radishes. A pita pocket stuffed with turkey, tomato, lettuce, and alfalfa sprouts. Snuggled in a sealed plastic bag, any of these make the perfect distraction—and they'll also guarantee you get your hard chew in. Another plus: With a good, solid, hard chew to chomp down on, who needs gum to pop those ears?

Finally, don't forget a bottle of water. Not only do planes dehydrate your skin and your body, but dryness can also upset your body's chemical balance. The water will help keep your system stabilized, your skin smooth, and jet lag at bay. True, you can most likely get bottled spring water on a plane, but why wait for the cart to come around when you can tote your favorite mineral water—and drink whenever you like?

"I Keep Wanting to Lose the Same Ten Pounds and I Can Never Do It. Why?"

I can't tell you how many times I've heard this. There are the technical reasons that can be fairly easily identified and corrected. These technical reasons should be the first place to look. Perhaps you're not clear about your "Extras." Maybe your portions are too big. Or maybe you're not exercising enough, so you're not metabolizing your food as efficiently as you could. Then again it could be the low blood sugar that comes from eating too big a meal—which makes you sluggish and unable to burn off your food. On the other hand, it could be that you are eating too *little*, since your metabolism slows down in order to conserve energy. And finally, these ten pounds could be proof that you are insulin-resistant.

Then again, there are the *fathead* reasons, the emotional reasons, why we can't lose those ten pounds—and even why we want to lose them in the first place! The most poignant example of what I call the "ten-pounds syndrome" was Samantha. She was beautiful, a former model who was now married with a young daughter. Most people would envy her figure, but Samantha only saw the ten pounds she had gained when pregnant. She already had a healthy exercise regime, one involving the Stairmaster, jogging, and ballet, and she leaped into the 5-Day Miracle Diet with enthusiasm.

At first all went well. Samantha slowly lost weight, one pound a week. But after losing six pounds, she began the "tease," forgetting hard-chew snacks, skipping breakfast, eating after dinner.

Realizing this had to be a *fathead* issue, I urged her to

talk about her feelings, but Samantha just kept saying she had to lose ten pounds. Period. She was extremely dogmatic in her thinking, as if those ten pounds were magical.

I knew they represented something more, and as it turned out, so did Samantha—eventually. She realized that the ten pounds were a great distraction from her life problems, in particular her need to put up a roadblock so that she wouldn't have to look for a better job, so that she wouldn't have to come to terms with her fear of success—and its underlying component of low self-esteem. ("I don't really deserve success, after all," she'd say.) Samantha never did lose those ten pounds. It didn't seem that important anymore, not after she got her promotion.

Ask yourself the questions I posed to Samantha. What do those ten pounds represent to you? Is there something else in your life that is bothering you, something that is too difficult to face? Remember, food can be a weapon of choice—and so can a need to diet.

After careful consideration, if you are still having problems with your "ten-pounds syndrome," I highly recommend asking your health professional for the name of a good therapist.

"Do I Need to Modify the Diet If I'm Menopausal?"

The 5-Day Miracle Diet is excellent for anyone at any age. It provides a healthy way to live your entire life. However, because menopause has been associated with calcium deficiency, I recommend increasing your supplement by 300 mgs. Also try to eat a variety of foods rich in calcium. Check the "Foods Rich in Calcium" list in chapter 3.

If your weight loss seems to be decreasing, say, only one-half to one pound a week or even less—and you are exercising regularly—I would consider *stripping the carbs* (see chapter 7) for one week to see whether the cravings stop and you feel better.

Many women in their forties and fifties who come to my office never had weight issues before menopause. I have found that their extra ten or twenty pounds drop off easily on the *stripping the carbs* diet.

I expect that more research will soon come out tying the hormonal fluctuations that occur in menopause with disruptions in the chemical process involved in good blood sugar.

"Will Your Diet Help Me with PMS?"

Absolutely! I have had countless clients tell me that their symptoms of PMS—their bloated feeling, moodiness, crampiness—all disappeared or greatly diminished on the 5-Day Miracle Diet. There's a reason for this: My program goes right to the endocrine system, the overall system that regulates your hormones. By eating the appropriate foods, you will supply the right nutrients to stoke the endocrine system that produces the hormones which will keep your body in balance, so the fluctuations that create PMS may not exist.

Blood sugar drops when you are premenstrual. Your entire endocrine system is gearing up for menstruation. Balanced blood sugar helps eliminate the emotional swings, while the regularity of the timed fruits and vegetables helps relieve the edema (or swelling) that occurs throughout your body and helps relieve the discomfort of enlarged breasts. It will alleviate some of the moodiness, too.

As with anything else, use the right materials, and you'll have a sound structure. If you're eating well, your body will be able to produce the right hormones and your chemistry will be on an even keel. It makes sense that by supplying the body with good food, you're giving it the ingredients to make a positive, healthy structure, which would alleviate the symptoms of PMS.

I like to use this analogy with my clients to illuminate the power of good blood sugar: A sweater is only as good as the raw materials you use. If you have a sweater that's made with 100 percent virgin wool, it's going to hold up better and longer than a sweater that's half polyester. The same goes for your body. If you feed it the right raw materials, it's going to perform much more efficiently. It, too, will hold up better and longer—for the *entire* month.

"How Can I Tell If My Fathead Involves Unconscious Impulses? If They're Unconscious, How Do I Find Them?"

Once my clients are in good blood sugar, we begin to delve into the *fathead* issues that might sabotage their weight-loss efforts. It's true that the clients who come to see me or call me on the phone have the benefit of "Adele Puhn" right there and on the case. But you, too, have me—within the pages of this book. Go back to chapter 5, which deals exclusively with *fathead* issues. Review your answers to the *fathead* quiz. Try to determine if your emotional need to eat is strongest when you're beginning to be successful in your weight-loss efforts or if the *fathead* seems intense right before a family function or if you find food a comfort and a stress-reducing aid when you are anxious, depressed, or overtired.

Here's another tip I give my clients: Close your eyes and imagine your "fantasy family." Don't feel inhibited. This is for your eyes and ears only. Try to imagine a family situation that makes you feel wonderful, secure, nurtured. Maybe it's your mother hugging you. Your father helping you with your homework. Your brother or sister returning the clothes/money/Game Boy he or she borrowed last year. Think of the expressions on your family's faces. See the love mirrored in their eyes, the smiles. See the comforting golden light. Imagine their conversation, their laughter, whatever.

Now open your eyes and ask yourself if this fantasy family is way out of reality. If so, you might be unconsciously trying to capture your fantasy, over and over again, with friends and within relationships. Since you never got what you needed as a child, you keep trying, as an adult, unconsciously and unsuccessfully to get what you want. You are still seeking what you never received. Since this is an irrational and unrealistic pattern, you will always be thwarted eventually—and perhaps resort to food as the way to keep your pain, your rage, and your sense of loss at bay.

This might sound a bit like psychobabble, but I assure you it is much more common than you might think. If imagining your fantasy family is painful, if it brings tears or denial, then you could very well be seeking to fill the void with food.

If this is your scenario, it has to be difficult—and painful—for you to address, especially alone. I strongly urge you to seek out a therapist to help you better understand and get beyond this particular *fathead* issue.

"Can I Eat Foods Not on Your Food Lists?"

Remember my refrain: You are practicing for maintenance from the moment you begin the 5-Day Miracle Diet. This is a lifestyle diet, not a temporary aberration until you go back to the way things were.

I remember Kate, an artist client with a fabulous sense of humor. She lost thirty-five pounds on my program. She exercised five times a week. She addressed her *fathead* issues head-on, using emotional food to feed the need for comfort and security. There seemed to be nothing that could stand in the way of her lifelong success. Indeed, she'd just received a lucrative assignment as a contributing editor to a fashion magazine.

Except . . . Without discussing the situation with me (she knew I'd quite rightly "burst her balloon" and show her the self-destructive reality of her behavior), she had a "larger plan." In her heart of hearts Kate had not changed. As soon as she lost thirty-five pounds, she decided that she was now a "thin person." She no longer had to diet. She could skip the articles about diets and fat in the magazines. She could eat what she wanted and enjoy every bite.

Basically she was right. As you well know by now, I insist that my clients eat what they want and enjoy every bite when they have their twice weekly "Food You Adore." But there's a crucial end to this sentence. Come on, you know it: *once you are in good blood sugar*.

The trouble with Kate is that she began to nibble, teasing herself with cookies and elaborate entrées. Her blood sugar plummeted and her apples and carrots disintegrated in the fridge.

The result? Kate gained back fifteen pounds and came back to see me. We began to examine what was going on inside her. She soon realized that she had to acknowledge the fact that she had to accept responsibility for her health and sense of well-being. Choosing a healthy lifestyle is not a death sentence. Like quitting smoking, such a choice is a positive affirmation of yourself, of what you believe in, and of your future.

Owning the 5-Day Miracle Diet means this is the way you eat most of the time, and less and less of the time you are *not* eating this way. The times you are *not* eating this way become the exceptions rather than the rule. When you own the program, you are going longer and longer periods without upsetting your blood sugar. It does not mean that suddenly, out of the blue, you've turned into Oprah Winfrey, Sharon Stone, Jimmy Smits, Susan Sarandon, Christie Brinkley, or Richard Gere. (And I guarantee that these celebrities are constantly on a "diet" regime. They have personal trainers, chefs who practice low-fat cooking, and a lifestyle that's filled with nonfood rewards.)

Some of my clients forget how they arrived here. Once on maintenance, they forget what they did—and what they accomplished. They forget that good blood sugar is their friend for life.

"Which Vitamins and Minerals Do I Need and Which Foods Have Them?"

The 5-Day Miracle Diet is the result of my many years of experience. I have researched the program and practiced it on myself and in my office, over and over again, refining it, defining it, and making it the compact, healthy, successful program it is.

If you follow my program, choosing foods from the lists I present in chapter 3, you will get a lot of the vitamins and minerals you need on a daily basis. Add a multi-vitamin-and-mineral and calcium-magnesium supplement for basic coverage. Each individual has his or her unique needs and should see a nutritionist for a comprehensive program.

I've also added a helpful list of vitamins and minerals found in various foods in appendix A. You can refer to this if you want more information.

And because all individuals are different, I once again urge you to see your health professional before starting this or any other diet program.

"My Friends Keep Saying, 'Enough Already!' I'm Beginning to Agree."

It's difficult to keep your eye on the prize when everyone around you is telling you you've already received it! Compliments are wonderful, and in an idealized world they'd just reaffirm your goals and make your resolve even stronger. Unfortunately saboteurs are always ready to pounce, and what greater *fathead* temptation than "Enough already." Yes, I've seen clients with images of chocolate truffles dancing in their head . . . dinner at eight at their favorite restaurant, bread basket and champagne already beckoning . . . pasta for lunch, pasta for dinner, even pasta for a snack!

Stop. Think. Identify and recognize your problem—and what the solutions are. Take the compliments in stride. Feel wonderful. Feel proud of yourself. But remember, owning the 5-Day Miracle Diet means you'll have it, always, like a supportive friend. Healthy eating and exercise do not mean you can never eat your chocolate truffles or your pasta. It just means making choices.

And if "enough already" is not quite at your goal, keep going. My maintenance program is waiting for you whenever you—and only you—have decided "enough already."

I've listed only twenty questions here. Perhaps you have others that you can't find answers for in this book. Remember, I'm here to help. I'm with you in spirit.

You're Not Going to Believe the Results

Oscar Wilde once wrote, "To love oneself is the beginning of a lifelong romance." In his clever statement lies a world of profound truth.

For some reason that love, that basic, primal, and extremely accessible love, is often the most difficult to embrace. We all have our ways of keeping that love at a distance, whether it be with weight, with self-doubt, or with actions that hurt rather than heal.

But love toward another must be preceded by this self-love. After all, if you can't love yourself, as the cliché goes, how can you love anyone else? And, taken another step, how can you believe anyone will love you back?

The 5-Day Miracle Diet is simply a program. It does not deal with hocus-pocus or mystical spells. The plan contains sound, scientific methodologies to keep food cravings at bay and help you lose weight and feel wonderful. But it is still only words *until you decide to implement them.*

And that's when the 5-Day Miracle Diet becomes more than "just a diet plan."

It becomes an act of love.

An act of affirmation.

Empowerment.

You have decided to do something positive about your life. You have made the choice to be healthy and live a life that is full and vital.

You, yes, you.

The miracle began when you bought this book, when you read through the program and the reasons why you eat the way you do, when you learned that you can fit this program into any lifestyle, in any time zone, in any social stratum. The miracle began with those first five days when you began to feel better than you ever have in your life. Suddenly there is that nudge of hope, that nudge that tells you that, after all these years, the reason you haven't stayed on a diet is not because you're not motivated, not because you're not strong enough, but because of your body's chemistry and the subtle ventriloquist called low blood sugar.

The hope then becomes more than a glimmer. You can see it. Yes, this time it will work. I can be healthy and full of energy. I can be thin.

I can make it work.

Me.

That's part of what my program offers you: a reason and a choice.

But there is one more thing I offer: love. A lifelong romance with *your* good health, *your* vitality, *your* strength. Quite simply, as I and thousands of my clients have discovered, the 5-Day Miracle Diet gives you the ability to love yourself.

And that more than anything else is the reason why this diet plan is a miracle.

To your new life.

To miracles.

To love.

> *With my warmest best wishes to you all,*
> Adele Puhn

APPENDIX A

Vitamins and Minerals
Found in Food

VITAMIN A (beta carotene)

Why we need it: For healthy tissues, skin, hair, and mucous membranes. Night vision. Vital for normal growth and reproduction.

Food sources: Yellow vegetables, such as winter squash, yams, sweet potatoes, and carrots. Dark green vegetables, such as broccoli, spinach, green beans, cabbage, and lettuce. Cantaloupe. Apples. Cauliflower. Pears. Cheese (no-fat and low-fat). Milk. Tofu. Egg yolks. Apricots.

VITAMIN B1 (thiamine)

Why we need it: Aids metabolism by helping to release energy from carbohydrates. Promotes healthy muscles and nerves, including central nervous system and heart. Helps fight fatigue and irritability.

Food sources: Meat, especially pork. Tofu. Whole-grain cereals, rice, and breads. Dried beans and peas, especially navy and black. Sunflower seeds. Nuts.

VITAMIN B2 (riboflavin)

Why we need it: Aids metabolic process by releasing energy from foods. Promotes clear vision, healthy hair, skin, and nails. Essential for growth.

Food sources: Chicken, turkey, and other poultry products.

All types of fish. Dried beans. Nuts. Sunflower seeds. Cheese (no-fat and low-fat). Eggs. Milk. Tofu. Plain yogurt. Whole-grain cereals, rice, and breads. Green leafy vegetables, such as spinach, broccoli, and cabbage. Seaweed.

VITAMIN B3 (niacin)

Why we need it: Creates efficient metabolism. Promotes healthy skin and hair. Important for healthy growth and maintenance of digestive tissue. Stimulates blood circulation.

Food sources: Veal. Pork products. Chicken, turkey, and other poultry. All types of fish. Nuts. Sunflower seeds. Dried beans, such as lentils and black-eyed peas. Leafy green vegetables, such as spinach, broccoli, cabbage, and lettuce. Whole-grain cereals, rice, and breads. Milk. Soy products. Eggs.

PANTOTHENIC ACID

Why we need it: Aids adrenal glands in producing proper amounts of hormones during stress. Promotes healthy skin, hair, and nerves.

Food sources: Nuts. All types of beans including kidney beans and lentils. Turkey, chicken, and other lean poultry products. Milk. Soy milk. Tofu. Tempeh.

VITAMIN B6

Why we need it: Helps metabolize fat. Aids body in breaking down protein to promote tissue growth. Helps liver release glycogen. Facilitates production of red blood cells. Helps regulate fluid balance in body.

Food sources: Sunflower seeds. All types of beans, including kidney and black beans and lentils. Lean turkey, chicken, and other poultry products. Leafy green vegetables, such as spinach, cabbage, broccoli, kohlrabi, and lettuce. All fruits and vegetables found on the 5-Day Miracle Diet.

VITAMIN B12

Why we need it: Facilitates production of red blood cells. Helps build genetic material in cells. Stimulates growth. Helps metabolize food. Promotes healthy nervous system.

Food sources: Red meat. Lean turkey, chicken, and other poultry products. Pork. Cottage cheese. Veal. Cheese (no-fat and low-fat). All types of fish, especially shellfish, such as lobster and shrimp. Milk. Soy milk. Tofu. Tempeh. Plain no-fat yogurt. Eggs.

BIOTIN

Why we need it: Helps metabolize food. Promotes efficient energy production.

Food sources: Found in almost every food in the 5-Day Miracle Diet, especially eggs.

FOLIC ACID

Why we need it: Facilitates production of red blood cells. Helps metabolize proteins. Vital during pregnancy for cell division.

Food sources: Green leafy vegetables, such as spinach, broccoli, cabbage, kohlrabi, and lettuce. All types of beans, including kidney and black beans, lentils, and chickpeas. Green beans. Whole-grain cereals, rice, grains, and breads. All fruits, including oranges, cantaloupe, apples, pears, and strawberries.

VITAMIN C

Why we need it: An essential vitamin for healthy teeth, bones, skin, and connective tissues. Helps heal bruises, bumps, and cuts. Stimulates the immune system. Aids the body's ability to absorb and use iron. An anti-oxidant that helps the body "claim" floating free-radical molecules that, if left loose, would help create premature aging.

Food sources: Citrus fruits, such as strawberries, oranges, grapefruit, and cantaloupe. Dark green vegetables, such as spinach, green beans, broccoli, kohlrabi, and kirbys. Cauliflower. Peppers (red, green, yellow, and purple). Tomatoes. Baking potatoes. Sweet potatoes. Pears. Apples. Carrots. Raw cabbage.

VITAMIN D

Why we need it: An essential vitamin for healthy teeth and bones. Helps regulate metabolism, especially when combined with dairy products.

Food sources: Skim milk. Soy milk. Nonfat plain yogurt. Cottage cheese. Cheese (no-fat and low-fat). Tofu. Tempeh. Tuna fish. Egg yolks. Fatty fish, such as salmon and sardines.

VITAMIN E

Why we need it: An antioxidant that helps the body "claim" floating free-radical molecules that, if left loose, would help create premature aging.

Food sources: Oil, including olive, canola, and safflower. Sunflower seeds. All types of fish and shellfish. Wheat germ. Whole-grain cereals, rice, and breads. Green leafy vegetables, such as spinach, broccoli, kohlrabi, and cabbage.

VITAMIN K

Why we need it: Essential for proper blood clotting.

Food sources: Green leafy vegetables, such as broccoli, kohlrabi, spinach, and cabbage. Cauliflower. Tofu.

CALCIUM

Why we need it: Essential for maintaining healthy bones, teeth, and muscles. Promotes normal blood clotting. Aids steady nervous system.

Food sources: Skim milk. Soy milk. Cottage cheese. Cheese (no-fat and low-fat). Tofu. Tempeh. Dark green leafy vegetables, such as broccoli, kale, and spinach. Beans, such as lentils, garbanzos, and peas. Sunflower seeds. Sesame seeds. Baked sweet potatoes. Beets. Nonfat plain yogurt. Mustard greens. Arugula. Fennel. Seaweed and kelp. All types of fish, especially scallops, shrimp, sardines, and salmon.

PHOSPHOROUS

Why we need it: Promotes healthy teeth and bones. Essential for production of genetic material, cell membranes, and enzymes used in metabolism and digestion. Aids proper metabolism.

Food sources: Red meat. Veal. Lean turkey, chicken, and other poultry products. All types of fish including salmon, trout, and cod. Skim milk. Soy milk. Cottage cheese. Cheese (no-fat and low-fat). Eggs. Sunflower seeds. Whole-grain cereals, rice, and breads. Wheat germ. Artichokes. Pears. All fruits and vegetables found on the 5-Day Miracle Diet.

MAGNESIUM

Why we need it: Promotes healthy bones. Helps regulate body temperature. Aids energy release from muscle storage. Essential for healthy cardiovascular system. Regulates mood. "Nature's tranquilizer."

Food sources: Whole-grain cereals, rice, and breads. Dark green leafy vegetables, such as spinach, kale, mustard greens, and broccoli. Sunflower seeds. All types of beans and legumes, including kidney beans and lentils. Tofu. Tempeh. All types of fish. Lean red meats. Lean turkey, chicken, and other poultry products. Unsweetened, natural peanut butter. Peaches. Nectarines.

SODIUM

Why we need it: Proper fluid balance. Healthy nervous system.
Food sources: All the foods on the 5-Day Miracle Diet supply sufficient daily sodium requirements.

POTASSIUM

Why we need it: Proper fluid balance. Vital for a healthy cardiovascular system. Healthy nervous system. Aids metabolism and proper energy release from foods.
Food sources: Found in all the foods on the 5-Day Miracle Diet. Especially bountiful in fruits, beans, vegetables, and lean meats.

CHLORIDE

Why we need it: Aids production of gastric juices. Necessary for proper digestion.
Food sources: All types of fish and shellfish. Skim milk. Soy milk. Cottage cheese. Eggs. Red meat. Veal. Pork. Lean turkey, chicken, and other poultry products.

IRON

Why we need it: Essential for red-blood-cell production, especially hemoglobin, which carries oxygen throughout the body. Promotes energy and healthy skin.
Food sources: Pork. Red meat. Whole-grain cereals, rice, and bread. All types of beans, including navy beans and lentils. Lean turkey, chicken, and other poultry products. All types of fish, especially clams. Beet greens. Mustard greens. Tofu. Walnuts.

COPPER

Why we need it: Helps promote red-blood-cell production, especially hemoglobin, which carries oxygen throughout the body. Aids healthy bones. Healthy nervous system. Healthy circulatory system.

Food sources: Whole-grain breads, cereals, and rice. Whole-wheat bread and cereal. Buckwheat. Shellfish. Walnuts. Sunflower seeds. All types of beans, including peas and lentils. Dark green leafy vegetables, such as kale, spinach, and broccoli. Prunes.

ZINC

Why we need it: Promotes hormonal secretion. Helps balance insulin production. Aids in blood formation. Promotes blood clotting. Keeps tissues healthy. Supports immune system. Healthy skin.

Food sources: Whole-grain breads, rice, and cereals, especially brown rice. Sunflower seeds. Lean turkey, chicken, and other poultry products. All types of fish and shellfish, especially clams and oysters. All types of beans, including navy beans and lentils. Lean red meat.

IODINE

Why we need it: Proper thyroid gland function.

Food sources: All types of fish and shellfish. Seaweeds, including kelp and nori. Cottage cheese. Skim milk. Soy milk. Cheese (no-fat and low-fat). Whole-grain breads.

FLUORIDE

Why we need it: Healthy teeth and gums.

Food sources: All types of fish and shellfish. Tea. Some waters (check labels).

CHROMIUM

Why we need it: Helps in production of energy. Helps in the metabolism of fat.

Food sources: Lean meat. All fish and seafood. Whole-grain cereals, rice, and breads. Lean chicken. Eggs.

SELENIUM

Why we need it: An antioxidant that helps the body "claim" floating free-radical molecules that, if left loose, would help create premature aging. Supports immune system.

Food sources: All types of fish and shellfish. Lean meats and poultry. Whole-grain cereals, rice, and breads. Onion and garlic.

MANGANESE

Why we need it: Stimulates enzyme activity.

Food sources: Whole-grain cereals, rice, and breads. All fruits and vegetables on the 5-Day Miracle Diet, especially spinach.

MOLYBDENUM

Why we need it: Stimulates enzyme activity. Promotes healthy teeth.

Food sources: All types of legumes and beans. Lean pork. Dark green leafy vegetables, such as spinach, kale, mustard greens, lettuce, and broccoli. Tomatoes. Skim milk. Whole-grain cereals, rice, and bread. Carrots. Winter squash. Wheat germ. Strawberries.

APPENDIX B

Blank Food Journal

DATE	/	/	/
DAY	MONDAY	TUESDAY	WEDNESDAY
BREAKFAST	TIME:	TIME:	TIME:
SNACK	TIME:	TIME:	TIME:
SNACK	TIME:	TIME:	TIME:
LUNCH	TIME:	TIME:	TIME:
SNACK	TIME:	TIME:	TIME:
SNACK	TIME:	TIME:	TIME:
DINNER	TIME:	TIME:	TIME:
COMMENTS			

/	/	/	/
THURSDAY	FRIDAY	SATURDAY	SUNDAY
TIME:	TIME:	TIME:	TIME:
TIME:	TIME:	TIME:	TIME:
TIME:	TIME:	TIME:	TIME:
TIME:	TIME:	TIME:	TIME:
TIME:	TIME:	TIME:	TIME:
TIME:	TIME:	TIME:	TIME:
TIME:	TIME:	TIME:	TIME:

A 10-Day Sample Food Journal

DATE	AUG/14	AUG/15	AUG/16
DAY	MONDAY	TUESDAY	WEDNESDAY
BREAKFAST	TIME: 7:15 tofu, 2 rye Wasas	TIME: 7:20 1 egg 1 slice toast water	TIME: 7:20 ½ c. cottage cheese 1 slice toast 9:00 coffee
SNACK	TIME: 9:00 apple, (See Adele—appt.)	TIME:	TIME: 9:30 pear
SNACK	TIME: 10:40 kirby	TIME:	TIME: 11:00 kirby
LUNCH	TIME: 12:30 lg. salad w. tomato, pepper (green), broc., cauli., 2 rice cakes, 3 oz. tuna. /Italian dressing	TIME: 12:15 lg. salad w. tomato, cauliflower, ½ c. cott. cheese, 2 rice cakes, balsamic vinegar, 1 pear	TIME: 12:00 lg. salad, cuke, 1 tomato, cauli., n.o. 3 oz. tuna 2 rice cakes, pepper
SNACK	TIME: 3:30 apple	TIME:	TIME: 4:00 apple
SNACK	TIME: 5:00 raw cauliflower	TIME: 4:00 yellow apple 5:00—kirby	TIME:
DINNER	TIME: 7:00 chicken (4oz.) stir-fry, veggies, olive oil	TIME: 7:10 bean soup lg. salad n.o. 1 tomato, cuke, 1 pepper	TIME: 6:30 4 oz. chicken, broccoli, steamed cauliflower
COMMENTS	Walked twice (power walks).	Period started. Felt great despite missing snacks.	CRASH!—binged on cookies tonight. Not eating snacks at right time—2 days in a row.

AUG/17	AUG/18	AUG/19	AUG/20
THURSDAY	FRIDAY	SATURDAY	SUNDAY
TIME: 7:15 1 egg 1 slice toast 1 c. coffee—all day!	TIME: 7:20 ½ c. cott. cheese 1 slice toast	TIME: 10:30 1 egg 1 slice toast coffee, water	TIME: 8:30 1 slice toast ½ c. cottage cheese 1 pear
TIME: 9:30 red apple	TIME: 8:45 red apple 1 c. coffee	TIME:	TIME:
TIME:	TIME: 11:15 carrots	TIME:	TIME: 10:30 (power walk)
TIME: 12:45 lg. salad, spinach, cauli., tomato, etc. 3 oz. tuna, balsamic vinegar, 2 rice cakes	TIME: 12:30 4 oz. salmon green beans steamed broc. & cauliflower, raw cauliflower	TIME: 12:00 lg. salad, raw veggies, 3 oz. tuna, 2 rice cakes, n.o.	TIME: 12:30 lg. salad w. tomato, veggies, 3 oz. tuna, 2 rice cakes (oil & vin.)
TIME: 3:00 green apple	TIME: 3:30 green apple	TIME: 2:00 green apple	TIME: 3:00 ½ cantaloupe
TIME: 5:00 carrots	TIME:	TIME: 4:00 carrots	TIME: 5:00 kirby
TIME: 6:30 marinara spaghetti, lg. salad w. spinach, cauli., tomato, pepper, lettuce, balsamic vinegar	TIME: 6:15 lg. salad, Tuscan bean soup, 1 c. veggie, ice tea	TIME: 6:00 lg. salad w. tomato, cuke, n.o., 6 oz. beef, broc., pepper, zucchini, tom.	TIME: 6:30 salad, n.o., tomato, 4 oz. chicken, oil, garlic, zuc., peppers, broc.
8:00—rice cakes. Still crashing! Rebound... from cookies yesterday, and missed 11:30 snack. Must do better tomorrow!	Coming back...	Hard! Needed too much protein at dinner, but still feeling better.	2nd walk after dinner!! I have so much energy.

DATE	AUG/21	AUG/22	AUG/23
DAY	MONDAY	TUESDAY	WEDNESDAY
BREAKFAST	TIME: 7:30 1 egg 1 slice toast decaf. water	TIME: 7:30 ½ c. cott. cheese 1 slice toast coffee	TIME: 7:00 1 egg 1 slice toast water
SNACK	TIME: 8:45 green apple (See Adele—appt.)	TIME: 8:45 pear	TIME: went back
SNACK	TIME: 10:30 carrots	TIME: 10:30 kirby	TIME: to sleep
LUNCH	TIME: 12:30 lg. salad, ½ tom./ ½ cuke, peppers, ½ c. cott. cheese, 2 rice cakes, vinegar	TIME: 12:50 salad w. tom, pepper, raw cauliflower, 3 oz. tuna, 2 rice cakes, n.o.	TIME: 1:00 salad with tomatoes, cauliflower, raw peppers, shrimp, 1 slice bread
SNACK	TIME: 3:00 strawberries	TIME: 2:45 strawberries	TIME: 4:00 pear
SNACK	TIME: 4:30 raw cauliflower	TIME: 5:00 carrots	TIME:
DINNER	TIME: 6:45 lg. salad w. tom., pepper, cauli., cuke. 1 c. couscous, n.o.	TIME: 6:30 mesquite chicken rice field salad baby asparagus	TIME: grilled portobello mushrooms, grilled salmon with dill, mix of green zucchini and summer squash
COMMENTS	Long stroll home! Feels amazing . . .	Got up early. Full of energy. Walked right past my favorite bakery without even realizing it! Enjoyed dinner.	Wow! Still have tons of energy. This really works.

Adele's Veggie Hints

By the time you finish reading *The 5-Day Miracle Diet*, you'll know that I'm passionate about vegetables. Yes, that's right. As passionate about vegetables as I am about cookies or champagne—but for different reasons.

I love vegetables because they do so much for me.

Hard-chew vegetables not only help control blood-sugar levels when eaten in the proper amounts at the proper time, but they are also chock-full of essential vitamins and minerals your body needs to function healthfully day after day.

Here are some hints to make your vegetables delectable, easy to munch, and, yes, even a passionate treat.

RAW-VEGETABLE HINTS

1. Buy a vegetable spinner. You'll be able to clean your vegetables in record time.
2. Make your salads ahead of time—using a large plastic bowl and cover. Buy a few heads of lettuce, say, Romaine, red-tipped, and arugula. Break them up and wash them. Spin them in your cleaner and pile the greens into your plastic bowl. All week, whenever you want a fresh green salad, you only have to open the bowl, grab a handful of greens, and voilà—salad.
3. Supermarkets and specialty stores now cater to health-conscious adults. Buy your hard chews already cut up

and ready to eat: broccoli florettes, baby carrots, cauliflower florettes, chopped red cabbage. You can even buy ready-made, prepackaged salads or, for real convenience, try the salad bar. (Since these veggies are not washed before cutting, it's essential you do so before eating.)

4. Experiment with different kinds of vegetables. Try that cute baby eggplant. Take a chance and buy some portobello mushrooms. Cut up some leeks into your salad. Broil an elephant garlic until brown. It's delicious. Garlicky, but not super strong.

COOKED-VEGETABLE HINTS

1. Grill slices of onion, eggplant, tomatoes, and zucchini in the broiler or on the grill. Brush lightly with olive oil and add seasonings of your choice. Cook until tender.

2. Prepare portobello mushrooms in your toaster oven. Simply sprinkle with crushed garlic and cook at 350 degrees until tender. Believe it or not, they actually taste like a luscious meat or fish steak!

3. Use fresh, ripe vegetables whenever possible. They might cost a bit more, but remember all the money you spent on frozen cakes, packaged cookies, and pints of ice cream?

4. Make raw vegetables more digestible, if necessary, by blanching them. Drop cleaned, ready-to-eat veggies in a pot of boiling water. Wait 1 or 2 minutes, then remove. Drop them into a bowl of ice water, then remove. The ice water stops the veggies from cooking and it sets the color so that you don't feel like you are eating yesterday's vegetables. They'll simply be a little bit softer and easier to eat.

5. Think vegetables as a sauce for pasta (at dinner

only!), rice, or couscous. They make a satisfying and fabulous meal. (And you'll swear it's fattening as you eat every bite.)

Here are a few recipes I've developed in my kitchen over the years. All of them have helped me love vegetables. I hope they'll do the same for you.

ADELE'S BEAN AND VEGETABLE DISH

Not quite chili, not quite sauce, this entrée is delicious served over couscous or rice. 4 servings

In a large saucepan, sauté:
1 tablespoon olive oil
2 cloves garlic, minced
1 large onion, finely chopped

When slightly brown, add:
2 8-oz. cans black beans
2 stalks celery, chopped
1 tablespoon chopped parsley
1 green pepper, chopped
Spices of your choice to taste (try coriander, herbes de Provence, or cilantro)

Simmer for 15 minutes, stirring occasionally.

Serve over rice.

ADELE'S CHUNKY VEGETABLE SAUCE

One of the reasons I love this sauce is its diversity. You can add just about any vegetables you have on hand. They all taste good when stirred with tomato and basil! This dish is also wonderful as a soup. Simply add more water and you have a warming soup on winter nights. Or pour on some dollops of Tabasco sauce and serve it cold for a variation on gazpacho. Another suggestion: Use this sauce on a baked potato. Yum! 4–6 servings

In a large saucepan on the stove, sauté:
2 cloves garlic, chopped
1 large onion, sliced

When translucent, add:
1 green pepper, chopped
1 stalk celery, chopped
1 medium zucchini, sliced
1 eggplant, cut into cubes
2 fresh tomatoes, roughly chopped
2 16-oz. cans peeled whole tomatoes (no sugar added!)
2 carrots, sliced
1 handful string beans, chopped
1 handful broccoli florettes, roughly chopped
½ cup water
3 tablespoons fresh basil, cleaned and chopped

Cover and simmer for 30 minutes, stirring occasionally. Add water if necessary. Season to taste before serving over pasta.

ADELE'S STUFFED EGGPLANT

I like to think of this recipe as rustic French. One-half eggplant makes a scrumptious vegetarian meal. You don't need any side dishes. Simply bring your knife and fork (and your bon appétit, of course!).

Preheat oven to 350°F.

Slice a large eggplant vertically, dividing it in half.
Prick the insides with a fork.
Place upside down on paper towels for 30 minutes. (This will get rid of any bitterness.)

Cook the eggplant in a skillet sprayed with vegetable oil on the stove for 20 minutes on low heat, or until the meat is tender.

While the eggplant halves are draining and cooking, cut the following vegetables into chunks and place in a large bowl:

1 medium zucchini
4 tomatoes, seeds removed
1 yellow pepper
1 green pepper
2 leeks
2 cloves garlic, minced
6 mushrooms

When the eggplants are ready, let them cool slightly.
When comfortable to handle, cut out the meat from the eggplant and chop it into chunks. Add to the bowl. You will be left with an eggplant "shell."

Add to the vegetables in the bowl:
¼ cup olive oil
¾ cup whole-grain bread crumbs or wheat germ
1 egg, beaten

Divide the contents of bowl in half and pour equal amounts in each eggplant shell.

Sprinkle the top with a bit more bread crumbs.

Sprinkle with some chopped no-fat Cheddar cheese.

Put in the oven for 30 minutes, or until the vegetables are tender when pierced with a fork and the bread crumbs are browned on top.

With a salad, makes a delicious one-dish meal for two.

ADELE'S ROAST VEGETABLE SUPPER

This dish fills a roasting pan with enough vegetables to be used as a side dish for 6 to 9 people. Add 1 cup of pasta or rice, potato or starchy vegetables (corn, winter squash, peas), or 2 ounces of cheese per portion and you have a quick and satisfying main dish.

Preheat oven to 350°F.

Place the following vegetables in a large bowl:
1 small head cauliflower, in florettes
1 medium zucchini, in ¼-inch slices
1 medium summer squash, in ¼-inch slices
1 cup string beans, chopped
1 red pepper, cut into chunks or rings
1 yellow pepper, cut into chunks or rings
2 medium carrots, cut in ¼-inch slices
8–10 cherry tomatoes
6–8 pearl onions, peeled
2–4 cloves garlic, peeled and diced

Bring to a boil in a medium saucepan:
1 can no-fat chicken broth or 1½ cans vegetable broth
½ teaspoon tarragon

½ teaspoon marjoram or savory
⅓ cup olive oil

Pour hot mixture over vegetables.

Put entire mixture in a roasting pan. Spread evenly. Cover with a lid or foil and bake for 1 hour, basting once or twice during cooking time.

Feel free to experiment with your own favorite vegetables or more exotic starches, such as couscous or lentils.

Sources

Almada, Anthony, "Sweet Talk and Bittersweet Truths," *Natural Healing*, March 1992.

Baar, Karen, "Time for a Fitness Pyramid? Extra Benefits from Exercise at Any Age," *The New York Times*, March 29, 1995.

Babayan, Suren, "Women May Have to Exercise Longer Than Men: Study," *Reuters*, August 24, 1995.

Beck, Melinda, et al., "The Losing Formula," *Newsweek*, April 30, 1990.

Brody, Jane, "Moderate Weight Gain Risky for Women, a Study Warns," *The New York Times*, September 14, 1995.

Califano, Julia, "Ready for the Runaway," *Heart & Soul*, June 1, 1995.

Chernin, Kim, *The Hungry Self: Women, Eating and Identity*, New York: Harper & Row, 1985.

Chisholm, Patricia, "Obesity Increases in U.S.," *Harvard Heart Letter*, vol. 5, November 1, 1994.

Colbin, Annemarie, *Food and Healing*, New York: Ballantine Books, 1986.

Ellis, Kenneth, "Body Composition, Obesity, and Weight Loss," *Journal of the American College of Nutrition*, vol. 13, no. 3, June 1994.

Etewiler, Donnell, "Give Yourself a Healthy Reward When You Achieve Goals," *Diabetes in the News*, vol. 13, November 1, 1994.

Giller, Robert M., M.D.; and Kathy Matthews, *Natural*

Prescriptions: Dr. Giller's Natural Treatments & Vitamin Therapies for More Than 10 Common Ailments, New York: Ballantine Books, 1994.

Goddard, Mary S., R.D., M.S.; Gloria Young, B.S., M.T.; and Robert Marcus, M.D., "The Effect of Amylose Content on Insulin and Glucose Responses to Ingested Rice," *The American Journal of Clinical Nutrition*, vol. 39, March 1984.

Heck, Traci, et al., "What Is Exercise Enjoyment? A Qualitative Investigation of Adult Exercise Maintainers," *Wellness Perspectives*, vol. 10, September 1, 1993.

Hirsch, Cheryl, "Blood Sugar and Brain Function," *Medical Nutrition*, Summer 1989.

Hollis, Judi, Ph.D., *Fat and Furious*, New York: Ballantine Books, 1994.

Jaret, Peter, "The Way to Lose Weight," *Health*, January–February 1995.

Jenkins, David, et al., "Nibbling Versus Gorging: Metabolic Advantages of Increased Meal Frequency," *New England Journal of Medicine*, vol. 321, no. 14, October 5, 1989.

Jenkins, Nancy Harmon, "Shopping for Rice Is No Longer a Simple Choice," *The New York Times*, March 29, 1995.

Kennedy, Carol, et al., "A Comparison of Body Image Perceptions of Exercising and Nonexercising College Students," *Wellness Perspectives*, vol. 11, April 1, 1995.

Nowlan, Mary Hegarty, and Elizabeth Hiser, "The Hungry Mind," *Eating Well*, May–June 1995.

O'Rahilly, S., et al., "Insulin Resistance as the Major Cause of Impaired Glucose Tolerance: A Self-Fulfilling Prophecy?" *Lancet*, vol. 344, August 27, 1994.

Rees, Michael, "Treat Obese Patients with Empathy and Emphasis on a Healthy Life-Style," *Modern Medicine*, vol. 63, July 1, 1995.

Rickabaugh, Tim, "If at First You Don't Succeed, Try Weight Loss Again and Again," *Diabetes in the News*, vol. 14, March 1, 1995.

Rippe, Dr. James M., with Karla Dougherty, *The Polar Fat Free and Fit Forever Program*, New York: Fireside, 1994.

Rippe, Dr. James M., and Ann Ward, Ph.D., with Karla Dougherty, *The Rockport Walking Program*, New York: Fireside, 1989.

Robb-Nicholson, Celeste, "Strength Training," *Harvard Women's Health Watch*, vol. 2, May 1, 1995.

Roth, Geneen, *Feeding the Hungry Heart: The Experience of Compulsive Eating*, New York: Signet, 1982.

———, *When Food Is Love: Exploring the Relationship Between Eating and Intimacy*, New York: Dutton, 1991.

———, *Why Weight? A Guide to Ending Compulsive Eating*, New York: Plume, 1989.

Shapiro, Laura, "Food Lover's Guide to Fat," *Newsweek*, December 5, 1994.

Shimer, Porter-Bean Adam, "Speedwork Speeds Fat Loss," *Runner's World*, vol. 30, April 1, 1995.

Smith, Barbara, Ph.D., "Sweet Addictions," *The Nutrition Report/Health Media of America*, vol. 12, no. 3, March 1994.

Smith, Sally, "The Great Diet Deception," *USA Today Magazine*, January 1, 1995.

Toufexis, Anastasia, "The New Scoop on Vitamins," *Time*, April 6, 1992.

Travis, J., "Mice Reveal Another Genetic Clue to Obesity," *Science News*, vol. 147, June 3, 1995.

Ulene, Dr. Art, *The Nutribase Guide to Carbohydrates, Calories & Fat in Your Food*, Garden City, N.Y.: Avery Publishing Group, 1995.

———. *The Nutribase Guide to Fat & Cholesterol in Your Food*, Garden City, N.Y.: Avery Publishing Group, 1995.

Williams, Bryan, "Insulin Resistance: The Shape of Things to Come," *Lancet*, vol. 334, August 20, 1994.

INDEX

Adele Puhn would like to hear from you. If the 5-Day Miracle Diet has brought "miracles" to your life, please write to:

*Adele Puhn, M.S., C.N.S.
c/o Nutritional Industries LLC
13 Cutter Mill Road
Suite 324
Great Neck, NY 11021*

Adele Puhn is available for lectures, seminars, and workshops based upon this book. Details will be sent upon request.

Here is the perfect companion to the diet that everyone's talking about—
because it works!

THE 5-DAY MIRACLE DIET COMPANION
by Adele Puhn, M.S., C.N.S.

You can boost the power of your own weight-loss miracle with...

- easy-to-use daily journal pages
- fact-filled weekly assessments
- inspiring monthly check-ins
- original mouthwatering recipes
- Adele's special tips on eating in your favorite restaurants
- solid advice for enjoying holidays and special occasions—while keeping weight off, too
- shopping with Adele—a pleasure, not a chore

Published by Ballantine Books.
Available in bookstores everywhere.

Coming in January 1998 from
Ballantine Books...

YOUR BODY BANK

**Getting Healthy and Staying
Healthy in Today's Toxic World**

by Adele Puhn, M.S., C.N.S.

A guide to finding and maintaining
a strong, healthy body, mind,
and soul.

Taking the mystery out of comple-
mentary medicine, Adele shows
how, when, and why to use
homeopathic herbs, remedies, and
supplements to live a healthier and
happier life—regardless of age or
current condition.